THE POLITICS OF SURVEILLANCE AND RESPONSE TO DISEASE OUTBREAKS

Global Health

Series Editor: Nana K. Poku,
Health Economics and AIDS Research Division (HEARD), South Africa

The benefits of globalization are potentially enormous, as a result of the increased sharing of ideas, cultures, life-saving technologies and efficient production processes. Yet globalization is under trial, partly because these benefits are not yet reaching hundreds of millions of the world's poor and partly because globalization has introduced new kinds of international problems and conflicts. Turmoil in one part of the world now spreads rapidly to others, through terrorism, armed conflict, environmental degradation or disease.

This timely series provides a robust and multi-disciplinary assessment of the asymmetrical nature of globalization. Books in the series encompass a variety of areas, including global health and the politics of governance, poverty and insecurity, gender and health and the implications of global pandemics.

Also in the series

HIV/AIDS and the South African State
Sovereignty and the Responsibility to Respond
Annamarie Bindenagel Šehović
ISBN 978 1 4724 2337 5

Living with HIV and Dying with AIDS
Diversity, Inequality and Human Rights in the Global Pandemic
Lesley Doyal with Len Doyal
ISBN 978 1 4094 3110 7

Informal Norms in Global Governance
Human Rights, Intellectual Property Rules and Access to Medicines
Wolfgang Hein and Suerie Moon
ISBN 978 1 4094 2633 2

Ethics and Security Aspects of Infectious Disease Control
Interdisciplinary Perspectives
Edited by Christian Enemark and Michael J. Selgelid
ISBN 978 1 4094 2253 2

The Politics of Surveillance and Response to Disease Outbreaks

The New Frontier for States and Non-state Actors

Edited by

SARA E. DAVIES
Queensland University of Technology, Australia

JEREMY R. YOUDE
University of Minnesota Duluth, USA

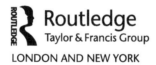
Routledge
Taylor & Francis Group

LONDON AND NEW YORK

First published 2015 by Ashgate Publishing

2 Park Square, Milton Park, Abingdon, Oxfordshire OX14 4RN
711 Third Avenue, New York, NY 10017

Routledge is an imprint of the Taylor & Francis Group, an informa business

First issued in paperback 2017

British Library Cataloguing in Publication Data
A catalogue record for this book is available from the British Library.

The Library of Congress has cataloged the printed edition as follows:
Davies, Sara Ellen.
  The politics of surveillance and response to disease outbreaks : the new frontier for states and non-state actors / by Sara E. Davies and Jeremy R. Youde.
      pages cm. -- (Global health)
  Includes bibliographical references and index.
  ISBN 978-1-4094-6718-2 (hardback)
  1. Public health surveillance--International cooperation. 2. Epidemics. 3. World health.
  I. Youde, Jeremy R., 1976- II. Title.
  RA441.D377 2015
  362.1--dc23

                                                                            2014030478

ISBN 978-1-4094-6718-2 (hbk)
ISBN 978-0-8153-7777-1 (pbk)

Contents

List of Figures and Tables

Figures

Tables

Notes on Contributors

Philip AbdelMalik, is Program Director in the Canadian Field Epidemiology Program at the Public Health Agency of Canada (PHAC).

Louise Boily, MA, is Senior Operations Manager in the Situational Awareness Section in the Centre for Emergency Preparedness and Response at the Public Health Agency of Canada (PHAC).

Richard Coker is Professor of Public Health, London School of Hygiene and Tropical Medicine, Visiting Professor at the Saw Swee Hock School of Public Health, NUS, Singapore, and Counselor to the Faculty of Public Health, Mahidol University, Bangkok. His research interest is in health systems and infectious diseases in SE Asia.

Nigel H. Collier is Marie Curie Research Fellow with the European Bioinformatics Institute in Cambridge, UK, and Associate Professor at the National Institute of Informatics, Japan and the Graduate University for Advanced Studies, Japan.

Sara E. Davies is ARC Future Fellow and QUT Vice Chancellor Research Fellow, Australian Centre for Health Law Research, Faculty of Law, Queensland University of Technology, Australia. She is also Program Director, Prevention of Mass Atrocities, Asia Pacific Centre for Responsibility to Protect (University of Queensland).

Jennifer S. Edge is Research Associate at Harvard Global Health Institute in the United States of America.

Steven J. Hoffman, BHSc, MA, JD, is an Assistant Professor of Clinical Epidemiology & Biostatistics at McMaster University in Canada and a Visiting Assistant Professor of Global Health at the Harvard School of Public Health in the United States of America.

Adam Kamradt-Scott is Senior Lecturer in the Centre for International Security Studies, Department of Government and International Relations, University of Sydney. Adam is also the Precinct Leader for the Humanities Node of the Marie Bashir Institute for Infectious Diseases and Biosecurity.

Richard Lemay is a Project Manager with the Centre for Emergency Preparedness and Response at the Public Health Agency of Canada.

Marco Liverani is a Lecturer at the London School of Hygiene & Tropical Medicine. He has worked on several aspects of infectious disease prevention and control, with a focus on Southeast Asia. Recent areas of interest include policy analysis and governance, risk assessment and management, and socio-economic aspects of disease emergence and transmission.

Abla Mawudeku, MPH, is Chief of the Centre for Emergency Preparedness and Response at the Public Health Agency of Canada (PHAC).

Simon Rushton is a Faculty Research Fellow in the Department of Politics at the University of Sheffield, and an Associate Fellow of the Centre on Global Health Security at Chatham House.

Theresa Seetoh is currently a management executive at the Ministry of Health, Singapore.

Frank L. Smith III is a Lecturer with the Centre for International Security Studies and the Department of Government and International Relations at the University of Sydney.

Clare Wenham is a PhD Candidate at the Centre for Health and International Relations, Aberystwyth University, Wales

Jeremy R. Youde is an associate professor of political science and department head at the University of Minnesota Duluth.

Acknowledgements

We sincerely thank the editors of *Global Public Health* and *Global Change, Peace and Security* for their support of the inclusion of some articles in this volume from the (respective) Special Issues we published with them.

Kirstin Howgate and Brenda Sharp, from Ashgate. Thank you for your endless support and patience. We would like to thank the anonymous reviewers for their insight and critique on the manuscript. The book is all the better because of these reviews. However, of course, responsibility for any errors lies with the Editors and contributors.

Our appreciation to the Centre for Governance and Public Policy, Griffith University, especially Professor Patrick Weller, for the financial and intellectual support provided for this project. A big thank you to Angela MacDonald for her assistance during and after the workshop 'Politics of Disease Surveillance', held in Brisbane, August 2011.

We would like to thank our families for their patience, support and love.

Sara E. Davies, Australian Centre for Health Law Research, QUT (Brisbane, 2014)
Jeremy R Youde, Department of Political Science, UMD (Duluth, 2014)

Introduction

A Study of the Politics of Surveillance and Responses to Disease Outbreaks

Sara E. Davies and Jeremy R. Youde

Infectious disease surveillance has become one of the cornerstones of global health politics in recent years. The International Health Regulations (2005) obligate member-states to make proactive, ongoing infectious disease surveillance one of their core functions, and the World Health Organization (WHO) has gained a certain global stature as the central repository of information in the face of disease outbreaks. This emphasis on surveillance has empowered new actors to take an active role in stopping the spread of pandemics, generated new technical means to identify potential pandemics as early as possible, and introduced significant debate over the meanings of terms like risk and human rights in the realm of public health. Despite all the rhetoric about the importance of infectious disease surveillance, the concept itself has received relatively little critical attention from academics, practitioners, and policymakers. What are the costs and benefits of extensive disease surveillance? How can it be effectively implemented, and what challenges prevent such implementation? What are the effects of allowing non-state actors to play an active role in a global governance process like disease surveillance? These are the sorts of questions we explore in this edited volume.

Global Health Governance and Disease Surveillance

In an analysis of the performance of global health governance initiatives, Ng and Ruger argue that one of the most striking features of the transition from international health governance to global health governance has been the continuation of the same "decades-old problems of insufficient coordination, the pursuit of national and organizational self-interest, inadequate participation by the recipients and targets of aid, and sheer lack of resources." They contend that diplomatic initiatives in the field of health are plagued, in particular, by a multiplicity of actors that have uncoordinated buy-in that affects and distorts the implementation (and sustainability) of these initiatives (Ng and Ruger 2011).

In 2005, a key moment in the global health governance initiative was the passage of the revised International Health Regulations (IHR) by the World Health Assembly. The revisions to this legal instrument, concerned with coordinating the prevention and containment of Public Health Emergencies of International

Concern (PHEIC), marked a conceptual and practical shift for the responsibilities of states, non-state actors and the World Health Organization. States were no longer only responsible for keeping outbreaks from entering their borders; they were also deemed responsible for preventing outbreaks spreading beyond their borders. Meanwhile, "informal" (non-state) actors and the WHO were given new responsibilities to, respectively, report outbreaks and (for the WHO) proactively seek state confirmation of outbreaks

Into this new environment, new "unofficial" disease surveillance networks have emerged. Disease surveillance networks are web-based networks that trawl the internet for news of infectious disease outbreaks and are primarily administered by non-state providers. For example, ProMED Mail was created in 1994 by the International Institute for Infectious Diseases and has been responsible for first reports of Nipah Virus in Malaysia (1998), H5N1 in Hong Kong (1997) and again in Thailand, Viet Nam and Indonesia (2004). There has been a proliferation of such networks since, including HealthMap, MediSys and BioCaster. These "unofficial" networks have the potential for tremendous power and impact on state behaviour, by virtue of the fact that they can report disease outbreaks without the prior permission of the affected state.

When the World Health Organization's first Director of International Health Regulations coordination, Dr Guénaël Rodier, gave an interview on the significance of the revised IHR (unanimously passed by the 2005 World Health Assembly) he was keen to stress their coercive power. Asked what were the incentives for states to comply with the revised IHR were, he replied:

> There are no police or fines here. There are, however, strong incentives for countries to comply. In today's information society, you cannot ignore or hide a problem for very long. You can perhaps ignore or hide an event for a day or two, but after a week it's virtually impossible. WHO and its partners have a powerful system of gathering intelligence that will pick anything up immediately ... One of the incentives for countries to report such events is that these will already have been reported via the electronic highway. We will be in a much better position to help if we have been involved early on by the affected country. The fear of being named and shamed by the media and other countries concerned by the situation is in itself an incentive. (Rodier 2007: 428)

Essentially, Rodier argued that the revised IHR embrace both normative and tactical changes. The revised IHR rest on states adopting a new norm under which states feel an obligation to their citizens and other countries to engage in active disease surveillance. States have a certain responsibility to themselves and each other, and will adhere to certain behavioural precepts to uphold this new understanding. Tactically, the growth and reliance on Information Communication Technology (ICT) fundamentally changes how public health and international organizations gather information on outbreak events through the media and blog monitoring—as much as if not more than, traditional communication from states. Disease intelligence-gathering entered the twenty-first century, it has been argued, while we were still in the twentieth century (Heymann and Rodier 2001). In particular, rather than waiting for states to inform WHO and other states of outbreaks, many chose to harness the technology to receive instant local media reports of outbreaks from all around the world, a technology that has been available from at least the mid-1990s (Grein et al. 2000; Brownstein et al. 2008).

However, the normative and tactical changes in the revised IHR do not just have coercive power, but the real potential to change the dominant picture of the state as the primary actor who determines their fidelity to international law according to their interests. If Rodier is correct, not only will states be forced to report against their interests, but their actual interests will change. The threat of exposure will become as crucial in informing a state's decision to report as the threat to the domestic economy.

As Carlos Castillo-Salgado (2010: 95) has argued, the dissemination of global surveillance information dates back to the mid-nineteenth century with state or state entities then agreeing to share reports of disease outbreak. However, the type of surveillance advocated in the new IHR "expands the efforts [of alert] to *prevent* and *control* the international spread of diseases with high risk of a global pandemic and any major public health risks." As such, the efforts required of states to proactively contain outbreaks and accommodate new actors in this endeavor of shared outbreak communication, as this book will detail, is novel.

These changing dynamics have called into question what exactly does global level disease surveillance—and the responses to these reports—demand from states and WHO in its contemporary manifestation post-IHR revisions. What sorts of technologies are available to anticipate and contain outbreaks? How useful are those technologies in resource-poor settings? How can surveillance systems accommodate reports from both state and non-state sources? What is the role of the WHO vis-à-vis the myriad of other national and international public health agencies in the world? What funding is available to support extensive disease surveillance systems? What do disease surveillance systems miss, and how do they fit into the broader array of public health activities?

In *Biopolitical Surveillance and Public Health in International Politics*, Youde explored how the individual human right to privacy had the potential to be eroded through the increased use of biosurveillance technology by governments and international organizations, such as WHO. This technology requires an almost inevitable intrusion into the behaviors, habits and interests of individuals—collecting data on individual entries into search engines, Facebook entries to individual travel history and purchases. This technology—and information on individual behavior—has become essential to provide a global public good that is expected by individuals and governments—infectious disease control (Youde 2009: 4). The book concluded that "the individual human rights standard needs to become a vital element of international infectious disease control programs" through ensuring that practice adheres to five core principles: transparency of surveillance practice, local engagement with surveillance technology, surveillance facilitates individual needs being met, surveillance is integrated into functioning public health systems, and there is a chance for appeal when rights and needs are neglected through surveillance or as a consequence of surveillance (Youde 2009: 178–87).

This question of global public goods—goods and services that accrue to more than one state and are non-rivalrous in their consumption and non-excludable in their enjoyment—has long plagued debates about the provision of global health services. Effective biopolitical surveillance must necessarily be non-rivalrous and non-excludable, but there exist significant questions as to whether surveillance is more of a luxury than a necessity for realizing some notion of a global "right to health." Do these innovations in disease surveillance represent progress toward realizing the "right to health," or do they take valuable resources and provide cover for reinforcing existing global health inequities?

In this book, we (Davies and Youde) employ five principles of infectious disease surveillance as a starting point to critically examine their utility for global surveillance programs and intergovernmental cooperation. We have asked contributors to assess how the reforms introduced by IHR (2005) demands new behavior, cooperation and responses from states, surveillance providers and international organizations; and, we have also asked the contributors to identify how these actors will accommodate the political impact and relationships required to facilitate outbreak alerts and response.

In July 2011, Griffith University sponsored a two-and-a-half day workshop that brought together academics, policymakers, and practitioners to critically examine what this new shared vision of infectious disease surveillance looks like, what challenges it faces, and what its future is. Hailing from the worlds of political science, public health, and information technology, the workshop sought to bring together constituencies that, unfortunately, do not always speak to or with each other. Many of the chapters in this book came from that workshop with a hope of continuing the conversations that began in Brisbane. We deliberately included a wide range of authors with unique and varying perspectives. This area remains relatively unexplored until now so we wanted the authors in this volume to defend their views on surveillance in examining the questions we post to them. We, as the editors, decided to keep the (slight) disagreements amongst the authors in their chapters so that the reader is not provided with a single unified view on disease surveillance. As such, we hope that each chapter can stand on its own and make a unique contribution to the debates on the theory and practice of biopolitical surveillance.

Plan of the Book

In this book we see the title, *The Politics of Surveillance and Responses to Disease Outbreaks*, as a statement and question. The technology available for surveillance networks—to trace outbreak events and report them publicly—is relatively new;

it appeared in the 1990s and really only gathered pace at the turn of the century (Hitchcock et al. 2007). We argue that there are five principles attached to this technology—transparency, local engagement, practical needs, integration and appeal (Youde 2009: 178)—that will illuminate what global surveillance is, how it works, who performs it, and what its political impact is.

In Chapter 1 we explore the transparency of the global surveillance system. Who are network surveillance actors and how do their infectious disease surveillance systems operate in the political environment? We (Davies and Youde) present the case that surveillance may be a technical exercise but it has political and human rights implications that states, surveillance systems and individuals need to be cognizant of when engaging and using these systems. In Chapter 2, Adam Kamradt-Scott and Simon Rushton provide a further investigation into the evolution and surveillance implications of the revised International Health Regulations (2005). They examine the expanded core capacity requirements attached to the revised IHR (2005) and how they have been fulfilled by states. Tracing the events during the H1N1 Swine Flu outbreak, they note how unofficial surveillance networks combined with WHO to create a normative expectation that states will report outbreaks. Endorsement of unofficial reporting forced states to realize that they had to participate or risk appearing inefficient and ineffective.

The use of global surveillance for local engagement is then explored in chapters 3 and 4. In Chapter 3, Theresa Seetoh and her colleagues examine how pandemic influenzas in different political settings (Thailand and the United States) in the past have been communicated to the public. They consider whether there is a global risk model that can be developed from these local experiences to allow for public awareness without public panic. They examine to what extent global surveillance networks can both hamper and assist local engagement in outbreak control.

As one attendee at the Brisbane workshop noted, an effective revised IHR requires "surveillance for action." Implementation gaps in surveillance technology, as discussed in Chapter 4, requires us to better understand the practical delivery of action expected from global surveillance under the revised IHR. In Chapter 4, Jeremy Youde conducts a compelling study of the IHR revisions and expanded surveillance capacity in the context of a fictional Zombie outbreak. He uses this case to illustrate how the human rights dimension of global surveillance and outbreak response remains under examined. There have been improvements in this area with the mention of human rights in the revised IHR (in the context of surveillance and quarantine), but he identifies a number of implementation gaps that, if ignored, at the local level would have real implications for infectious control and the population at large.

Implementation gaps in surveillance technology, as discussed in Chapter 4, requires us to better understand who is presently conducting global surveillance, and how does their work integrate with local health systems and political environments? In chapters 5 and 6, we look at the contributions from a variety of key global disease surveillance systems that are currently under operation. In Chapter 5, Abla Mawudeku, Director of Global Public Health Information Network with Public Health Agency of Canada, and her colleagues, present the (relatively recent) history of global disease surveillance, noting that despite much of the technology is still in development it has been remarkably influential in changing state behavior and expectations concerning knowledge of disease outbreaks. The most dramatic outcome Mawudeku et al. identify is the shift in expectations concerning surveillance and reports of novel outbreak events—concern is no longer on will an outbreak be reported—but on refining the technology to collect the right information as soon as possible. In Chapter 6, Nigel Collier—creator of BioCaster, a text-mining tool that provides "epidemic intelligence" by analyzing social and news media on the Internet concerning the Asia-Pacific region—explores the function and power of such technology for changing the behavior of individuals and states in response to disease outbreaks. Collier examines the impact that the use of social media tools will have on epidemiologic intelligence, the shortfalls of this technology in areas where there are technological "black holes" due to capacity and/or political constraints, and the ultimate changes that this technology will bring to the surveillance practices of states.

The final section of the book explores the grounds where controversies may arise concerning the development and use of global disease outbreak surveillance. Biopolitical surveillance does not exist within a vacuum, and its successes and failures interact with the larger political environments. In Chapter 7, Clare Wenham begins with a critical examination of the future of global health surveillance amongst states and international organizations, specifically WHO. She explores the unique surveillance role that WHO promoted, in cooperation with GPHIN Canada, and the outbreak response practices that WHO promoted in the development of Global Outbreak Alert Response Network (GOARN). WHO strongly promoted the global value of these intelligence-gathering tools in the SARS outbreak and during the drafting of the IHR (2005) revisions. WHO sought, and has received, much attention when a disease outbreak alert is issued from its system. However, Wenham identifies that with the evolution of global surveillance and outbreak response, WHO has been increasingly pushed out of the technical management of these alerts—by both states and alternative surveillance providers. This exclusion, Wenham argues, may risk WHO's long-term influence on states regarding outbreak information sharing and response.

In Chapter 8, Frank Smith explores how the global surveillance system engage with local health systems in the specific case of H5N1 Avian Influenza outbreak in Indonesia. He finds the global system wanting and argues for a more critical analysis of the revised IHR and the outbreak reporting requirements attached to the instrument. He notes that surveillance performance may be improving but states are perhaps more determined than ever that the enhanced surveillance capacity does not diminish their sovereign authority over virus samples and intrusion of WHO into outbreak investigations.

In Chapter 9, Youde examines the United States' National Strategy for Biosurveillance (NSB), released by the Obama administration in 2012. The strategy presents a unique case in which a sovereign state has explicitly integrated biosurveillance into its overall operational strategy. NSB offers the possibility for creating a well-integrated, comprehensive biosurveillance system that draws on resources at all levels and facilitates communication among relevant actors. At the same time, Youde suggests the heavy emphasis within NSB on detecting potential bioterror agents and emphasizing the military's role in biosurveillance may suggest that NSB's mandate will be more limited.

Finally, Jenny Edge and Steven Hoffman take these same issues of properly implementing an effective biosurveillance strategy at the local level and look for common themes. They identify common shortcomings among national governments that limit the possibility of a comprehensive global biosurveillance strategy operating effectively at the local level, but they also argue that hope is not lost. Their suggested strategies for strengthening biosurveillance systems increase the likelihood that such systems can effectively respond to our collective ability to respond to future epidemics.

Disease surveillance faces significant obstacles in terms of information sharing, building technical capabilities, and agreeing to common definitions. In the conclusion we explore the obstacles and benefits of global disease surveillance. IHR (2005) significantly reordered the global health governance architecture, and the effects of its innovations continue to be felt. While keeping such cautions in mind, we argue that there exists for the most part international engagement in moving forward with the necessary changes to ensure that all people can benefit from the advances in disease surveillance. But such engagement requires understanding that to fulfill the needs of all five principles—transparency, engagement, practical use, integration and appeal—requires focusing on global surveillance not just as an act of technology, but a political act with political consequences. Global surveillance, not unlike biosurveillance, requires politically attuned surveillance principles to improve the practices and the receptiveness of states.

References

Brownstein, J.S., Freifeld, C.C., Reis, B.Y., and Mandl, K.D. 2008. Surveillance sans frontières: Internet-based emerging infectious disease intelligence and the HealthMap project. *Public Library of Science* Medicine, 5 (7): 1019–24.

Grein, T.W., Kande-Bure, K.O., Rodier, G.R., et al. 2008. Rumors of disease in the global village: Outbreak verification. *Emerging Infectious Diseases*, 6 (2): 97–102.

Heymann, D.L. and Rodier, G.R. 2001. The WHO Operational Support Team to the Global Outbreak Alert and Response Network, "hot spots in a wired world: WHO surveillance of emerging and re-emerging infectious diseases." *Lancet Infectious Diseases*, 1 (5): 345–53.

Hitchcock, P., Chamberlain, A., Van Wagoner, M. et al. 2007. Challenges to Global Surveillance and Response to Infectious Disease Outbreaks of International Importance, *Biosecurity and Bioterrorism*, 5 (3): 206–27.

Ng, N.Y. and Ruger, J.P., 2011. Global health governance at a crossroads. *Global Health Governance*, 4 (2): 1–37.

Rodier, G.R. 2007. New rules on international public health security. *Bulletin of the World Health Organization*, 85 (6), 428–30.

Youde, J. 2009. *Biopolitical Surveillance and Public Health in International Politics*. New York: Palgrave Macmillan.

Chapter 1

Surveillance, Response, and Responsibilities in the 2005 International Health Regulations

Sara E. Davies and Jeremy R. Youde

Introduction

When the World Health Organization's (WHO) first Director of International Health Regulations (IHR) coordination, Dr Guénaël Rodier, gave an interview on the significance of the revised IHR (unanimously passed by the 2005 World Health Assembly) he was keen to stress their coercive power. Asked what were the incentives for states to comply with the revised IHR, he replied:

> In today's information society, you cannot ignore or hide a problem for very long. You can perhaps ignore or hide an event for a day or two, but after a week it's virtually impossible. WHO and its partners have a powerful system of gathering intelligence that will pick anything up immediately ... One of the incentives for countries to report such events is that these will already have been reported via the electronic highway. We will be in a much better position to help if we have been involved early on by the affected country. The fear of being named and shamed by the media and other countries concerned by the situation is in itself an incentive. (Rodier 2007: 428–30)

Essentially, Rodier argued that the revised IHR embrace both normative and tactical changes—but its real power is intelligence gathering. The revised IHR rest on states adopting a new norm under which states feel an obligation to their citizens and other countries to engage in active disease surveillance. States have a certain responsibility to themselves and each other, and will adhere to certain behavioral precepts to uphold this new understanding. The combination of the growth and reliance on information communication technology (ICT) and recognition of the importance of respecting human rights in disease surveillance fundamentally changes how public health and international organizations gather and act on information on outbreak events. The media, blogs, and SMS messages work in tandem with recognition of human rights to monitor disease outbreaks, and have become as important, if not more so, as traditional communication from states.

As early as 2000, public health surveillance was evolving from a government-controlled tool to one that individuals could harness and control. Rather than wait for states to inform WHO and other states of outbreaks, individuals and non-government organizations have been encouraged to harness this technology to instantly relay local media reports of outbreaks around the world (Grein et al. 2000, Brownstein et al. 2008). Between 1997 and 2001, approximately two-thirds of reports about infectious disease outbreaks initially came through these new sources rather than official country reports (Heymann et al. 2001: 352). The revised IHR encourage states to report outbreaks and respect human rights for fear of being named and shamed if they fail to do so—the technological capacity of individuals to contribute to global outbreak surveillance is changing, in turn, what states are expected to survey and report.

We propose that the revised IHR, in particular its inclusion of the WHO's right to receive non-state surveillance reports and the inaugural reference to international human rights principles in outbreak response, has a significance that may go beyond outbreak response. States have increasingly associated their capacity to respond to outbreaks with their responsibility as sovereign states in an international society. The failure to respond in a timely manner to an infectious disease outbreak is increasingly shameful for a "responsible" state, which as we further detail below, has the potential to either enrich or curtail the rights of individuals during and after an outbreak event.

Most analyses of the revised IHR and the new obligations they introduced have primarily concentrated on the relationship between the state and WHO, or the strength of the structures—between the state and WHO—to comply with the IHR. Neglected in these analyses, though, is an examination of whether the revised IHR's emphasis on surveillance has empowered a new actor—the individual. In this chapter, we ask how the inclusion of ICT and human rights principles into the revised IHR has empowered the individual. We interpret the "empowerment" claim as being one that could apply in a number of ways—from the individual providing disease outbreak alerts, to states introducing quarantine law the reflects the need for disease containment but is responsive to the individuals rights of citizens and non-citizens. Most of all, in this chapter, we are interested in the concept of sovereignty as responsibility that was promoted within the revised IHR. The revised IHR allowed non-state reports and made explicit reference to human rights instruments, we propose, because governments were persuaded that responsible states allow individuals to seek responsive and effective outbreak response from their states. Further, if a state fails to uphold this obligation within the revised IHR, then individuals have the right to take the means to "name and shame" them. There still exist significant limitations on the ability of individuals to fully realize their potential with regards to ICT and human rights recognition, as we will discuss in this chapter. Despite such shortcomings, we propose—and the contributions that follow in this book further reveal in the areas of surveillance, outbreak containment, timely reporting and risk communication—that significant advances have been made under this revision. The question is whether there exists the potential to further this nascent attempt at realizing sovereignty as responsibility in the area of outbreak surveillance, response, and containment.

In this chapter we focus on two key elements that were introduced in the revised IHR that directly engage the role of the individual as much as the state and the WHO: recognition of human rights principles in outbreak response, and the allowance for non-state actors to directly communicate with WHO and share outbreak surveillance intelligence. We explore the political impact of these two developments in four sections. First, we define how the concept of global biosurveillance developed under the revised IHR and how this definition delineates the decision making process in IHR (2005) that spells out the situations in which states, non-state actors, or individuals should report disease outbreaks to WHO. Second, we examine how IHR (2005) empowers individuals through recognizing and respecting human rights. Third, we look at the ability of the individual to report and access information about disease outbreaks through information communication technology (ICT) systems. Finally, we present the present the existing shortcomings and ambiguities in the IHR (2005)'s relationship between the individual, the sovereign, and the international community.

Health Surveillance and the IHR (2005)

Public health surveillance—the capacity to do it promptly, accurately, and on an ongoing basis—has developed a very specific significance within global health politics (Weir and Mykhalovkiy 2010). In 2005, the World Health Assembly passed Resolution 58.3, which defined surveillance as:

> The systematic ongoing collection, collation, and analysis of data for public health purposes and the timely dissemination of public health information for assessment and public health response as necessary. (WHO 2005)

Particularly important here is the emphasis on collecting information to guide action. The data gathered through public health surveillance are important only in that they facilitate appropriate responses. This change was particularly important given how the revised IHR shifted its surveillance and reporting mandates.

Chapter 2 provides more detail on the changes embodied within IHR (2005) and the reasons behind its significant reforms, but it is useful to highlight some of the rationale at this point. At the most fundamental level, the IHR had to be reformed because they were no longer relevant to the health challenges the international community faced. IHR (1969) relied on passive surveillance mechanisms that focused only on very specific diseases and offered no opportunity for non-state actors to play any role. What little surveillance did occur only targeted points of entry and exit, thus leaving most of any given country (and its citizens) undefended and irrelevant to the IHR's reporting mechanisms.

By the last decade of the twentieth century, it was clear that new and re-emergent infectious diseases simply could not be addressed by the IHR. States saw a need for a more active form of biopolitical surveillance in order to find new disease outbreaks and stop them as soon as possible. The growth in the number of reputable and reliable nongovernmental organizations, combined with the recognition that states may have motivations not to report disease outbreaks, encouraged consideration of the role non-state actors could play in addressing health security as we entered the twenty-first century.

IHR (2005) fundamentally transformed health surveillance in four key ways. First, it introduced the concept of the "all-risks" approach to surveillance. Instead of specifying specific diseases or conditions that would trigger surveillance mechanisms, the "all-risk" approach focused on "public health emergencies of international concern" (PHEIC). Such events threatened the international community, had the opportunity to spread, and required international cooperation to adequately address. Gone was the list of notifiable diseases from IHR (1969). In its place was a decision-making matrix to allow state and non-state actors to assess whether they needed to report an outbreak to WHO (see Figure 1.1). Second, IHR (2005) also set up permanent surveillance and reporting structures. A state had to constantly remain vigilant for outbreaks, and it always had to have a direct line to WHO in case of a reportable outbreak. Third, IHR (2005) gave WHO permission to accept and act on reports from non-state sources. This ended the bottleneck that, in the past, had allowed states to hide potentially embarrassing information about outbreaks and stymied WHO's ability to act. Finally, the new International Health Regulations placed human rights at the core of responding to public health emergencies of international concern. Governments had to always remain cognizant of the human rights implications of any actions they took to stop a disease's spread. If a state introduced limitations on human rights to combat an outbreak, such action had to be justified, minimal in its application, and limited in its duration. This put IHR (2005)'s mandates in line with 1985's Siracusa Principles, which explicitly lays out the narrow conditions under which governments can temporarily abrogate human rights (United Nations 1985).

These four changes to IHR (1969) are so far-reaching and removed from the scope in its predecessor that calling the changes "revisions" understates the enormity of the changes. The 2005 instrument—through the expanded scope and surveillance obligations, and the inclusion of an expanded reporting system and human rights principles—embodies multiple technical and legislative changes by the state to meet their core capacity requirements to the instrument. We contend that the revised IHR incorporates a deeper understanding of what a responsible sovereign should do in the event of an outbreak. This understanding is particularly notable, as we will present next, through the portioning of power to the individual under the IHR in the areas of human rights recognition and outbreak reporting. Both inclusions are potential avenues for individual agency that, theoretically, allows a person to challenge the behavior of a state in the event of an outbreak according to the IHR specified chain of events. Of course, these inclusions are far from perfect, but their presence is a notable advance to the concept of sovereignty as responsibility in the area of outbreak surveillance and response.

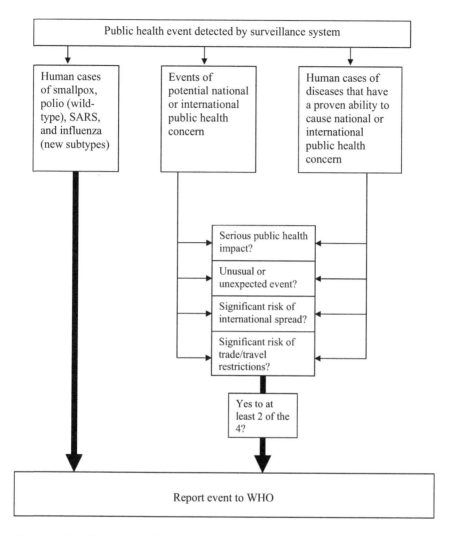

Figure 1.1   Decisionmaking instrument for IHR (2005), adapted from Annex 2

Human Rights in IHR (2005)

Between the IHR's original incarnation and its 2005 revised version, public health officials came to recognize the importance of human rights in implementing effective disease control strategies. Six articles within IHR (2005) address human rights. Article 3 states that IHR (2005) should be implemented "with full respect for the dignity, human rights, and fundamental freedom of persons." Article 23 states that travelers should not be subject to medical examinations without their consent and that any such examinations should be as minimally invasive as possible. Article 31 reaffirms Article 3, specifically highlighting the importance of respecting travelers' dignity, human rights, and fundamental freedoms. Article 42 states that the IHR (2005) should be implemented in a transparent, non-discriminatory manner. Article 43 guarantees to states the right to implement their own disease control measures outside the formal IHR (2005) process, provided that they are generally consistent with IHR (2005) and not more intrusive than necessary. Finally, Article 45 states that personal data is kept anonymous and confidential, and it be retained only as long as necessary for its specific purpose.

IHR (2005)'s emphasis on human rights adds a useful counterweight to the increased surveillance measures that are promoted as a core capacity requirement for states to meet their IHR obligations. More surveillance for more diseases and from more sources may engender suspicion and anger, but IHR (2005) provide the suspicious with an out. They know they have certain rights that must be respected, and the state knows that it must respect those rights. The Regulations provide the aggrieved with a framework for demanding their rights. All parties understand what the state owes its citizens and travelers within its borders. IHR (2005) offer "explicit protections of the interests of individuals" (Plotkin 2007: 841)—something completely absent from previous versions.

IHR (2005) recognize the importance of human rights by expanding public health surveillance beyond the state. National government officials may lack the awareness of disease outbreaks, or they may have incentives for concealing that information. Non-governmental organizations, local health clinics, local media sources, and individuals seeing changes in their communities may be better positioned to witness and understand that a problem is emerging. It can take time for information to trickle up to national health officials in the old passive surveillance systems. The more proactive, diffuse surveillance encapsulated in IHR (2005) streamlines the process of getting necessary information to WHO in a timely manner. The explicit inclusion of non-state actors in an international treaty represents a significant step forward. Non-state actors and individuals, through social media, can help ensure that states live up to their international legal obligations.

IHR (2005) and Internet-based Surveillance

The World Health Assembly (WHA) formalized the role of internet-based surveillance when it passed Resolution 54.14 in 2001, thus greatly expanding individual access to reporting systems. This resolution gave WHO the authority to incorporate internet surveillance and reporting programs (ISRPs) into its efforts to verify outbreaks and offer assistance with infection control, diagnostics, and fieldwork teams to afflicted states through its Global Outbreak Alert and Response Network (GOARN) (Heymann et al. 2001). While WHA Resolution 54.14 does not specifically mention GOARN or any particular ISRPs, their work was documented in the report of the WHO Secretariat (A54/9)—and Report A54/9 and WHA54.17 were both presented during the same WHA session (WHO 2001).

The underlying premise of GOARN and its associated Global Public Health Intelligence Network (GPHIN) is that "reports of infectious disease events around the world are regularly received by WHO through formal laboratory and epidemiological channels and from sources such as nongovernmental organizations, the media or electronic discussion groups." GPHIN provides the conduit to "seek, collect and verify information on reported epidemics, working closely with its collaborating centers, governments and governmental agencies, as well as relevant nongovernmental organizations and other partners in the global outbreak alert and response network" (WHO 2001: paragraph 7–8).

Despite falling under the innocuous label "Other Reports," Article 9 of the revised IHR introduced far-reaching changes in disease reporting procedures. Under this article, states authorized the WHO to take into account "sources other than [official] notifications or consultations" and required it to "assess these reports according to established epidemiological principles and then communicate information on the event to the State Party in whose territory the event is allegedly occurring" (WHO 2005: Article 9.1). Furthermore, the article mandates that states respond to WHO communications within 24 hours while allowing the *source* of the report to remain confidential. This may not be of paramount importance for ISRPs (depending on the ISRP source, media or informant), but it is for the nongovernmental organizations, religious organizations, or individuals who can also inform WHO of outbreak events.

During the 1990s, the evolution of internet technology inspired the creation of "global" surveillance networks. Some of these internet surveillance networks, such as BioCaster (see Chapter 6), rely primarily upon ontology software for text mining and language translation for report compilation. Others, such as GPHIN (see Chapter 5), rely on analyst software and human analysts. Under GPHIN, analysts with language proficiency in Arabic, Farsi, English, Spanish, Russian, Chinese, Portuguese and French sift through thousands of reports produced daily to determine which ones need to be placed on the subscriber-only alert page. GPHIN was one of the first real-time surveillance networks created, developed in cooperation with WHO Headquarters with Public Health Agency of Canada in 1996. Its reports are primarily issued to fee-paying subscribers and are therefore not publicly accessible. HealthMap is a free access internet surveillance network that analyses media reports on a scale similar to GPHIN and also collates reports from other surveillance internet providers such as MedISys (EU joint research center project), ProMED Mail, WHO and Google Search Term Trends—including blogs and "social media" sites—to produce real-time alerts of disease outbreak with color codes indicating source reliability (which entails "last minute" human moderation prior to posting) (Castillo-Salgado 2010).

With the wide range of internet surveillance networks, questions arise about the accuracy and value of the reports they produce (Hartley et al. 2010). Many argue that these networks are vital to the global disease reporting alert and response structure. GPHIN has been essential to the WHO's capacity to identify disease events and provide direct assistance to states, sometimes prior to those states and their neighbors, being aware of the extent of the outbreak (Heymann et al. 2008). As Pat Drury, head of Alert and Response Operations at WHO Headquarters, argued to the United Kingdom's (UK) Intergovernmental Organizations Select Committee in 2008, such "sources of information" help WHO's special operations center identify which media and incident reports need to be assessed for risk to the local and international community, which leads to recommendations for the country and WHO to take appropriate action (House of Lords 2008: 211). For example, WHO was able to use local reports of higher than usual pneumonia outbreaks in Southern China over 2002–2003 to seek clarification of the event, which turned out to be SARS. Similarly, online discussions on the ProMED Mail site among witnesses in China enhanced the risk assessment process at WHO Headquarters, informing their decision to request permission from the Chinese government to dispatch an investigation team in February 2003 to enter China to verify the extent of the outbreak (Heymann and Rodier 2004: 173–5; Madoff and Woodall 2005). The fact that it was less likely that states would be able to prevent the leakage of information about disease outbreaks, given the proliferation of internet surveillance networks, and that states were able to find the "signal" amongst the "noise" (Brownstein et al. 2008: 1019), was one of the key reasons why they agreed to IHR (2005) revisions that provided for WHO (2005) under Article 9 to "take into account reports from sources other than notifications or consultations and shall assess these reports according to established epidemiological principles and then communicate information on the event to the State Party in whose territory the event is allegedly occurring."

Ambiguities and Underdevelopment in the IHR (2005)'s Global Health Nexus

The recognition of human rights and the empowerment of non-state sources to contribute to epidemic infectious disease outbreaks are both hallmarks of IHR (2005). By including both of these elements, IHR (2005) sought to make sovereigns accountable for their health outbreak response at both the global and individual level by empowering individuals (O'Malley et al. 2009). Surveillance has become a political act in that it signifies a states responsibility to report IHR listed diseases, irrespective of capacity.

Despite these lofty goals, success has been more mixed in practice and the politics is complicated. The rhetoric supporting these dramatic changes to better incorporate the individual into these global practices did not necessarily translate into the appropriate activities. This is not to suggest that IHR (2005) is fatally flawed or that the underlying principle—sovereigns as responsible actors in outbreak response—is merely utopian wishful thinking. Instead, these difficulties reflect that existent oversights and ambiguities undermine the IHR's ability to live up to its promises. Bringing attention to them and shaming states that fail to live up to their obligations, though, will allow for changes and improvements.

Falling Short on Human Rights

The revised International Health Regulations' explicit embrace of human rights represents a significant step forward in infectious disease surveillance. By acknowledging the importance of respecting human rights, IHR (2005) can allay some of the fears that may exist around disease surveillance systems. The inclusion of human rights-related clauses also reflects the changing norms and standards within the global community.

Despite this progress, though, the force of human rights protections in IHR (2005) is underdeveloped and lacking in substantial backing. Chapter 2 details these shortcomings in greater detail, but it is important to acknowledge here that IHR (2005) conceptualizes human rights in a highly ambiguous manner. It is unclear *whose* human rights should be respected, as many of the explicit references to human rights exist in reference to travelers as opposed to residents or citizens. Furthermore, IHR (2005) does not reference any existent human rights treaties, depriving the regulations of firm precedents for understanding and implementing human rights protections. There is also no mechanism for investigating human rights abuses within WHO. While IHR (2005) call on states to respect human rights, they designate no office or agency to take action if one or more of those states fail to uphold their human rights obligations.

Being more explicit about human rights protections within IHR (2005) would encourage states to better integrate human rights thinking into their application of the Regulations. There is scope for WHO to clarify how states may fulfill their responsibilities towards the IHR in a way that does not abrogate or ignore the potential for individuals to contribute to, and benefit from, the IHR in an emancipatory way. But WHO has a delicate balance to tread here. Beyond the self-monitoring tool, there remains a gap between promoting human rights in the IHR and how the Organization may engage in some measure of monitoring or investigation of reports of human rights violations. The IHR (2005) Review Committee advocated WHO consult with state authorities when media reports suggested that human rights violations occurred (WHO 2011: 82). This arrangement would presumably be less formal than an actual investigation of human rights violations—something WHO lacks the resources or experience to conduct on its own—but even an informal approach could still signal to states that their actions do receive notice. As Chapter 2 goes on to reveal, it is on this latter point where unofficial sources can perhaps play their most useful role in encouraging compliance with and respect for human rights within health surveillance procedures.

Limitations in Internet-based Surveillance

Internet-based health surveillance systems should give individuals greater access to disease outbreak reporting systems, especially when governments may have an interest in censoring or selectively releasing information about disease outbreaks to the public's detriment. While this holds great promise, the experiences thus far suggest that these internet-based surveillance systems continue to give governments and official news sources a dominant voice. Individuals have less access than originally hoped for, and the systems themselves struggle to distinguish between official government and individual reports.

When we are attempting to track the efficiency, effectiveness and coverage of surveillance technologies—whether at the national or global level—we need to understand more about the political systems in which these technologies are operating. A quick scan of a MedISys or HealthMap output for 30 days will generate a lot of news media sources, but the vast majority of their content has been informed by public health officials releasing outbreak news. Governments may also spread rumors in order to advance their own interests (Brownstein et al. 2008: 1022), and Blench demonstrated that the quantity of official report sources—which are verified—is virtually equal to that of news media report sources (Blench 2010: slide 19). As Nigel Collier notes in Chapter Six, the epidemic intelligence upon which internet-based surveillance systems rely still struggle to figure out how to deal with the possibility of bias in their data. If these systems are using potentially biased information from official sources, this may inadvertently compromise or weaken their efficacy. Despite its important implications, the basic fact that at least half of all the reports come from the government itself has not yet penetrated discussion about the utility of surveillance for keeping governments transparent and how to test the quality of surveillance reports from governments during an outbreak (Heymann et al. 2008; Rodier 2007; Klobentz 2010: 122–3).

Understanding that governments are a significant source for ISRPs is important for two reasons. First, failure to acknowledge this fact feeds into the potentially unwarranted notion that states are not cooperating with the release of health information. Second, this neglect of the government's role as a source of information inflates the "intelligence" capacity of ISRPs without acknowledging their success relies upon governments making this information available. Therefore, what is new and needs to be emphasized is the search tool that ISRPs provide and the promotional impact of this information for people in situations where information cannot break through the state barrier. We cannot know precisely to what extent ISRPs are ahead of states until there is a clearer distinction in the ISRP reporting of outbreaks between sources that have some level of associated government input and those that are wholly "independent," which in turn "shames" states to engage in higher quality surveillance and response.

Noting the source limitations of servers also allows us to realistically understand the contribution that individuals and ISRPs can make to shedding light on those places where the communication and political freedom to report is constrained. HealthMap has argued that while 85% of its reports come from news media sources, there is a "clear bias towards increased reporting from countries with higher numbers of media outlets, more developed public health resources, and greater availability of electronic communication infrastructure" (Brownstein et al. 2008: 1021). The French Institute for Public Health Surveillance has noted similar concerns about the coverage gaps that their server has in particular geographic locations, and GPHIN has also referred to such coverage gaps (Rotrueau et al. 2007: 1591, Blench 2008: 299–303). Surveillance "blackholes" also arise in locations that place limits on the freedom of the internet, press, and independent actors. Previous experiences detailed by Madoff and Woodall (2005) reveal that it is highly unlikely individuals in autocratic countries would be able or willing to make extensive use of such internet technology. Nor can we assume that the provision of anonymity will make it any easier for the NGOs on the ground in countries where they are strictly bound to memorandum of understandings with their host government (i.e. North Korea) and where access to the internet is limited, monitored or regulated. There is not much that ISRPs or WHO can do about these problems, but heightened awareness of the human rights implications of "early reporting" and ISRP monitoring of such deficiencies, may facilitate more individual risks to supply those early warnings and constrain the retaliatory response of the state against that individual. In sum, there needs to be further consideration of how civil liberties and political freedoms are deeply connected to the efficiency of ISRPs and health system performance in general.

There can be no doubt that the allowance of non-state communications to WHO of a suspected outbreak heralds an important moment for situating power and agency beyond the nation state. We need to understand, though, how instances of individual agency work before we start proclaiming its transformative potential. First, there remain profound limitations for communicating outbreaks in despotic, autocratic regimes without the political or civil freedoms to freely communicate. The fact that there has been such little discussion of this, and especially the practical implications of the confidentiality clause under IHR (2005), is cause for concern (Youde 2009).

Second, we need to acknowledge the role of the state in assisting Article 9, and how it influences the work of ISRPs specifically. The study by Emily Chan and her colleagues, for example, noted that within the vast majority of reports on sites such as ProMed, HealthMap and MedISys, many of their online updates include government representatives reporting outbreak events or confirming the existence of ongoing tests to determine source or type of outbreak (Chan et al. 2010). Rarely is it acknowledged that the ISRP may have found an outbreak that the state already knew existed, furthermore that the ISRP found it because the *state reported the event*. In sum, the view is that the public airing of the "signal"—rather than who issued the signal—creates the impetus for action, but this view is flawed if the signal came from the state in the first instance.

Conclusion

As the chapters that follow in this volume will reveal, the revised IHR has presented a significantly new expectation on the responsibility of the state and the wider international community concerning disease outbreak surveillance. Instead of being solely a top-down process driven entirely by state interests, IHR (2005) now functions as the nexus that mediates the states responsibility to the individual and the global community. The treaty aims to link the individuals affected by its biosurveillance requirements with the policymakers who set up these systems. In this way, it aims to empower individuals by explicitly recognizing the important role of human rights in devising a global health regime and by harnessing the power of information communication technologies to allow individuals to share and access information about the infectious disease outbreaks that could potentially affect them.

While the revised IHR shows some promise, the treaty remains underspecified and ambiguous in certain crucial areas. As such, the promises of human rights and the ability of individuals to make meaningful contributions to reporting infectious disease outbreaks have not yet met expectations. This does not mean that we are failing to see sovereignty as responsibility in action—the acceptance of the IHR revisions confirms this point—but it does mean that we cannot rest on our laurels. Just as global health is an ever-changing field, so too our analysis of technological innovation, the action that improved surveillance facilitates (and demands), along with the expectations of effective sovereign policy commitment to this responsibility must all change and adapt. Most crucially, it must be recognized that surveillance may not be a political act but it engages with political actors, political situations and has political repercussions.

References

Blench, M. 2008. *Global Public Health Intelligence Network (GPHIN)*, 8th AMTA Conference, Hawaii, 21–25 October 2008, Available at: http://www.mt-archive.info/AMTA-2008-Blench.pdf [Accessed: 10 October 2011].

Blench, M. 2010. *Global Public Health Intelligence Network (GPHIN)*. [Online: Global Risk Forum]. Available at: http://www.slideshare.net/GRFDavos/idrcdavosmediumppt [Accessed: 10 October 2011].

Brownstein, J.S., Freifeld, C.C., Reis, B.Y. and Mandl, K.D. 2008. Surveillance Sans Frontières: Internet-Based Emerging Infectious Disease Intelligence and the HealthMap Project. *Public Library of Science Medicine*, 5 (7), 1019–24.

Castillo-Salgado, C. 2010. Trends and Directions of Global Public Health Surveillance. *Epidemiologic Review*, 32 (1), 93–9.

Chan, E.H., Brewer, T.F., Madoff, L.C., et al. 2010. Global Capacity for Emerging Infectious Disease Detection. *Proceedings of the National Academy of Sciences*, 107 (50), 21701–6.

Grein, T.W., Kande-Bure, K.M., Rodier, G., et al. 2000. Rumors of Disease in the Global Village: Outbreak Verification. *Emerging Infectious Diseases*, 6 (2), 97–102.

Hartley, D., Nelson, N., Walters, R., et al. 2010. Landscape of International Event-based Biosurveillance. *Emerging Health Threats Journal*, 3 (3), 1–7.

Heymann, D.L., Rodier, G. and WHO Operational Support Team to the Global Outbreak Alert and Response Network. 2001. Hot Spots in a Wired World: WHO Surveillance of Emerging and Re-emerging Infectious Diseases. *The Lancet Infectious Diseases*, 1 (5), 345–53.

Heymann, D. and Rodier, G. 2004. Global Surveillance, National Surveillance and SARS. *Emerging Infectious Diseases*, 10 (2), 173–5.

House of Lords. 2008. *Diseases Know No Frontiers: How Effective are Intergovernmental Organisations in Controlling their Spread? Volume II: Evidence*. Select Committee on Intergovernmental Organizations, 1st Report Session of 2007–08, HL Paper 143–II. London: The Stationery Office Limited.

Klobentz, G.D. 2010. Biosecurity Reconsidered: Calibrating Biological Threats and Responses. *International Security*, 34 (4), 96–132.

Madoff, L.C. and Woodall, J.P. 2005. The Internet and the Global Monitoring of Emerging Diseases: Lessons from the First 10 Years of ProMed-Mail. *Archives of Medical Research*, 36 (6), 724–30.

O'Malley, P., Rainford, J. and Thompson, A. 2009. Transparency during Public Health Emergencies: From Rhetoric to Reality. *Bulletin of the World Health Organization*, 87 (8), 614–18.

Plotkin, B.J. 2007. Human rights and Other Provisions in the revised International Health Regulations. *Public Health*, 121 (11), 840–45.

Rodier, G. 2007. New Rules on International Public Health Security. *Bulletin of the World Health Organization*, 85 (6), 428–31.

Rotrueau, B., Barboza, P., Tarantola, A. and Paquet, C. 2007. International Epidemic Intelligence at the Institut de Veille Sanitaire, France. *Emerging Infectious Diseases*, 13 (10), 1590–92.

United Nations. 1985. *Siracusa Principles on the Limitation and Derogation Provisions in the International Covenant on Civil and Political Rights*, UN Document E/CN.4/1985/4, Annex. Available at http://www1.umn.edu/human rts/instree/siracusaprinciples.html [accessed 22 May 2014].

Weir, L. and Mykhalovkiy, E. 2010. *Global Public Health Vigilance: Creating a World on Alert*. London: Routledge.

WHO 2001. *Global Health Security—Epidemic Alert and Response* [Online: Fifty-Fourth World Health Assembly, Geneva, Switzerland]. Available at: http:// apps.who.int/medicinedocs/documents/s16357e/s16357e.pdf [Accessed: 16 July 2011].

_____. 2005. *Revision of the International Health Regulations (2005)* [Online: Fifty-Eighth World Health Assembly, Geneva, Switzerland]. Available at: http://www.who.int/gb/ebwha/pdf_files/WHA58/A58_4-en.pdf [Accessed: 8 July 2011].

_____. 2011. *Implementation of the International Health Regulations (2005): Report of the Reporting Committee on the Functioning of the International Health Regulations (2005) in Relation to Pandemic H1N1 (2009)* [Online: Sixty-Fourth World Health Assembly, Geneva, Switzerland]. Available at: http://www.ghd-net.org/sites/default/files/A64_10-en.pdf [Accessed: 26 July 2011].

Youde, J. 2009. *Biopolitical Surveillance and Public Health in International Relations*. New York: Palgrave Macmillan.

Chapter 2

The Revised International Health Regulations and Outbreak Response

Simon Rushton and Adam Kamradt-Scott

Introduction

By its very nature, public international law frequently conflicts with, and impinges upon, state sovereignty. Indeed it is intentionally designed to do so, its purpose being to regulate the behaviour of states in the international system by codifying certain rules, principles and expectations, and enshrining them in treaties, guidelines and legal agreements. Over time the scope of public international law has expanded dramatically. Policy areas previously considered 'domestic' have come to be subject to international law, with the consequence that, as Neff has noted,

> There scarcely seemed any walk of life that was not being energetically "internationalized" after 1945 – from monetary policy to civil aviation, from human rights to environmental protection, from atomic energy to economic development, from deep-sea bed mining to the exploration of outer space, from democracy and governance to transnational crime-fighting. (Neff 2003: 54)

Moreover, as globalizing processes have progressively encouraged greater interconnectedness, the demand for codified international rules appears to be growing rather than diminishing.

The application of public international law to cross-border health issues is not, however, a new development. There have long been attempts, prompted by concerns over communicable disease outbreaks hampering international trade, to establish frameworks to guide interstate cooperation, although it has not always been easy in practice for states to reach an agreement. In 1851, in response to the worldwide spread of cholera and the severe impact it was having on the populations and international trade of European powers, the first International Sanitary Convention was held in an attempt to establish some consistent rules around quarantine practices. The meeting, which was mostly attended by European governments, failed to achieve its objective. Despite another 14 meetings and conventions being held over the next 100 years, it was not until the creation of the World Health Organization (WHO) in 1948, and the passage of the International Sanitary Regulations in 1951, that a universal agreement was eventually reached.

When adopted in 1951, the International Sanitary Regulations, renamed the International Health Regulations (IHR) in 1969, applied to six 'quarantinable' diseases (WHO 1951; 1983). Under the terms of the agreement, WHO member states were expected to report outbreaks of these six diseases and, where necessary, to take certain actions to prevent their importation from other affected territories. Over time, the number of diseases subject to the IHR was progressively reduced so that, by 1981, the IHR applied to only three – cholera, plague and yellow fever. Nonetheless, from the time of their entry into force the IHR suffered from a lack of compliance, primarily because governments, concerned over their reputation and/or the trade restrictions that other countries would impose, often declined to report outbreaks. At the same time, states often responded to outbreaks in other countries by implementing disproportionately severe travel and trade restrictions, further undermining the likelihood of states seeing it as in their interests to report outbreaks in future. In 1995, the decision was taken to revise and update the IHR, principally to broaden the scope of diseases subject to the Regulations but also to address the pervading lack of compliance. The 58th World Health Assembly (WHA) subsequently endorsed a new version of the Regulations in May 2005, and the new legislative framework officially entered into force on 15 July 2007.

This chapter examines one particular aspect of the revised IHR (referred to hereafter as IHR (2005)): the 'additional health measures' that states are permitted to implement in the event of a Public Health Emergency of International Concern (PHEIC). As already noted in Chapter 1, these provisions were specifically designed to address one of the key shortcomings of 1951 and 1969 IHR; namely, the imposition of disproportionate travel and trade restrictions on states reporting outbreaks, and as such go to the heart of the IHR's overall aim of offering protection against the international spread of disease 'in ways that are commensurate with and restricted to public health risks, and which avoid unnecessary interference with international traffic and trade' (WHO 2008: 10). As we argue in this chapter, these new provisions, which have been formally adopted by states as part of IHR (2005), represent a significant change to the normative framework that underpins global health security. The expectations the new rules place on states are substantially different, and the degree to which the authority to determine the appropriateness of particular measures has been ceded to WHO has real implications for notions of state sovereignty that effectively constitute a new norm. Whilst the new norm clearly builds upon the rules under previous versions of the IHR, in many ways it is qualitatively different. In the context of surveillance, as will be discussed below, what is particularly significant about the revised IHR reference to outbreak reporting is the expectation that outbreak surveillance and response is a practice that all states (regardless of capacity) should be doing.

This chapter, which proceeds in three parts, seeks to assess the extent to which this new international norm has been internalized by the WHO's member states. It first provides a brief outline of the changes relating to trade and travel-related additional health measures under IHR (2005) and identifies the content of the new norm. In the second section, the chapter sketches out a social constructivist understanding of international norms and how they affect state behaviour, in particular looking at the 'internalization' process through which norm-compliant behaviour becomes routinized within states' practices, albeit with the possibility of non-compliance remaining. Social constructivists argue that most states abide by international norms most of the time, and tell us that certain things can be expected on those occasions when states do not comply, including that the noncompliant state will usually attempt to justify its actions and that other states can be expected to criticise its behaviour. Accordingly, constructivists would argue, the presence or absence of these elements can give us important insights regarding the extent to which states have been socialized into a new norm. Whilst it is beyond the scope of this chapter to rigorously test this constructivist framework against other theoretical explanations for compliance and deviance, we argue in the chapter's third and final section that the discourse around the actions of certain countries during the 2009 H1N1 pandemic – and in particular the justifications for, and criticisms of, their behaviour – suggests that the constructivist case is at least a plausible one and, what is more, is suggestive of the existence of a widely shared international norm. We conclude by discussing what the discourse over H1N1 suggests about the extent to which the new norm concerning additional health measures has been internalized by states.

The IHR 2005 and 'Additional Health Measures'

The history of the revision of the IHR – a process which began in 1995 and was concluded in 2005 – has been discussed in considerable detail elsewhere (Fidler 2005; Kamradt-Scott 2010). It is not our intention, therefore, to revisit that history here. It is notable, however, that the vast majority of attention to date has been focussed upon the outbreak reporting requirements that IHR (2005) place on states. Here we focus instead on the development of another norm that has been enshrined within the revised Regulations, namely the expectation that, when confronted with a public health risk or PHEIC, states will adhere to the advice of WHO and will not, in seeking to prevent the importation of disease into their territory, take any action that may cause unnecessary or unjustified harm to international travel and trade.

Put another way, under the terms of IHR (2005), member states have agreed to place limits on their sovereignty, restricting the range of actions they may legitimately take in responding to public health risks and PHEICs. Although they do remain free to take any action designed to protect human health, as outlined in various articles throughout the revised framework – notably Articles 15–19 and 43 – governments have agreed to abide by WHO's recommendations in responding to disease outbreaks and, importantly, to not exceed that advice except where a clear public health rationale and justification for doing so exists. Where governments do decide to diverge from WHO advice and implement so-called 'additional health measures' that are more restrictive, invasive, or intrusive than

WHO recommends, under Article 43 of the revised IHR they are now required to provide WHO with a justification for their actions and to present scientific evidence in support of their case. As we will show below, whilst earlier versions of the IHR did contain articles which addressed travel and trade measures, the scale of the changes – in particular the shift in authority from states to WHO – is so significant as to constitute a genuinely new international norm that places significant constraints on the sovereignty of member states.

Two contextual explanations are important in the case of additional health measures. The first is that they are crucial to meeting the IHR's overall objective of providing the maximum security against the international spread of infectious disease whilst causing the minimum possible interference with international trade and traffic. Striking this balance had been central to every precursor of IHR (2005), from the International Sanitary Conventions of the nineteenth century through to the 1969 version of the IHR, and was seen as no less important for the new regulations. Indeed, given the centrality of a globalized economy and international free trade to contemporary international relations, the importance of this balance for the success of the new Regulations was arguably even greater. In recognition of this, WHO went to great lengths to address the compatibility of the IHR with existing trade agreements, such as those under the World Trade Organization. The second important aspect to highlight is that the excessively stringent measures put in place by some states in response to disease outbreaks under the previous (1969) version of the IHR were one of the problems that the revision process sought to overcome. Economically damaging overreactions to disease outbreaks were frequently cited as one of the reasons why governments refused to report such events. Cash and Narasimhan (2000), for example, showed how the economic losses resulting from trade restrictions imposed as a result of cholera and plague outbreaks in Peru and India respectively served as real disincentives for states to report disease outbreaks.

Previous versions of the IHR did limit the scope of legitimate health measures, but the rules changed significantly in the latest IHR. The 1969 version of the Regulations contained a number of specific provisions to this effect, including prohibitions on refusing entry to ships and aircraft not infected (Article 28) and on a state applying health measures to a ship that does not call at one of its ports (Article 32). As Barbara van Tigerstrom (2006) has noted, many of these provisions were narrowly defined and focussed on the limited number of diseases that were notifiable under IHR (1969). The 2005 version of the IHR includes a number of similar provisions that limit the measures that states may implement, some of which derive from the 1969 version. Article 25, for example, limits the measures that can be applied to ships and aircraft in transit; Article 26 does the same for lorries, trains and coaches in transit; Article 27 addresses the measures states can take in relation to an infected conveyance; and Articles 28 and 29 deal with ships, aircraft, lorries, trains and coaches at ports of entry.

In more general terms, however, what has occurred in IHR (2005) is a shift away from 'an approach which prohibited all measures save those specifically authorized by the regulations, and moved towards a set of restrictions based on certain principles (e.g. the need for scientific evidence, and the use of the least restrictive measures reasonably available) and procedures (e.g. notifying WHO of additional measures, and reviewing every three months)' (van Tigerstrom 2006: 53–4). It is these new general principles and procedures that, for us, constitute a new international norm that has the effect of constraining state sovereignty in significant ways. The expectations on state behaviour – the very heart of a 'norm' – have altered dramatically.

Under Articles 15 and 16 of IHR (2005) the WHO Director-General has been imbued with the authority to issue recommendations to member states on appropriate health measures in the event of a PHEIC. Article 18(2) outlines the types of recommendations that can be made in respect of trade restrictions thus:

> Recommendations issued by WHO to States Parties with respect to baggage, cargo, containers, conveyances, goods and postal parcels may include the following advice:
> * no specific health measures are advised;
> * review manifest and routing;
> * implement inspections;
> * review proof of measures taken on departure or in transit to eliminate infection or contamination;
> * implement treatment of the baggage, cargo, containers, conveyances, goods, postal parcels or human remains to remove infection or contamination, including vectors and reservoirs;
> * the use of specific health measures to ensure the safe handling and transport of human remains;
> * implement isolation or quarantine;
> * seizure and destruction of infected or contaminated or suspect baggage, cargo, containers, conveyances, goods or postal parcels under controlled conditions if no available treatment or process will otherwise be successful; and
> * refuse departure or entry. (WHO 2008: 17–18)

States are generally expected to follow whatever recommendations the Director-General announces. Article 43 does allow states to impose measures beyond what the Director-General advises (and even to impose measures specifically prohibited under other Articles), but only if those actions:

> are otherwise consistent with these Regulations. Such measures shall not be more restrictive of international traffic and not more invasive or intrusive to persons than reasonably available alternatives that would achieve the appropriate level of health protection. (WHO 2008: 29)

In deciding whether or not to introduce additional health measures states are required to take into account:

a. scientific principles;
b. scientific evidence that there is a risk to human health, or where such evidence is lacking, the available information including from the WHO, other relevant intergovernmental organizations, and international bodies; and
c. any available guidance or advice from the WHO (WHO 2008; Article 43, para. 2).

Upon receipt of this information, the WHO is authorized to share this data with other governments and assess the appropriateness of the measures taken. Where the organization deems that there is insufficient cause to justify the state's actions, WHO is again authorized to comment on this publicly, and to request the government in question to reconsider the measures. Although IHR (2005) does not allow for WHO to impose penalties on those states that do not comply, by publicly requesting that the state reconsider its actions – in effect granting the WHO the ability to 'name and shame' – the organization's authority as an independent arbiter has been substantially reinforced. What we have in terms of trade restrictions and disease control under IHR (2005), therefore, is a general principle that any restrictions should be the minimum necessary to provide for health security and an expectation that the Director-General will offer guidance on appropriate restrictions in the event of a PHEIC. But the provisions authorize states to go beyond these recommendations *only* if they can justify doing so on the basis of scientific evidence.

This new norm emerged during the Intergovernmental Working Group's negotiation of the IHR revisions, a lengthy process that began in the 1990s, but it was given new impetus following the SARS outbreak of 2003. As evidenced by the many textual amendments and proposals to early draft versions of the revised IHR framework, the norm was debated extensively throughout the intergovernmental negotiations. In adopting IHR (2005), which the World Health Assembly unanimously endorsed in 2005, though, all member states formally consented to the new norm, and to the new constraints it placed on their sovereignty, in order to benefit from collective efforts to achieve global health security. The questions that subsequently arise, however, are: to what extent states can now be expected to comply with that commitment, and whether the record of (non)compliance to date can shed light on the extent to which the norm has been internalized.

Compliance and Non-compliance: Insights from Social Constructivist Theory

Thus far we have described the new approach to additional health measures as an international norm, and social constructivists argue that the behaviour of states within international society is regulated by such norms, whether they are 'soft' behavioural expectations or 'hard' international law (Finnemore 2000). States can and do violate norms, but the degree of compliance – even on the part of the most powerful states in the international system – tends to be higher than rational choice theorists predict. Indeed, constructivists claim, it is this tendency to comply with international norms that makes the continued functioning of an international society of states possible (Wendt 1992). Where a state does violate the rules of international society it will usually feel compelled to provide the other members of that society with some justification for its actions. This justification may take any one of a variety of forms: claiming that the rule does not apply to the particular circumstances in question; arguing that the action is in line with the conflicting requirements of a different norm; claiming that the circumstances are so exceptional as to make non-compliance an acceptable course of action; or, most fundamentally, arguing that the norm is not a valid rule of international society. In general, constructivists would argue, states tend not to undertake actions that cannot be legitimated by reference to the prevailing law, rules and norms of international society, and they tend to behave for the most part in ways that are prescribed by international norms.

That said, it is important not to overestimate the extent to which state behaviour is determined by international norms. Just as is the case with domestic law, states are able to violate widely-held international norms, frequently with little or no prospect of any 'punishment' being imposed. The constructivist response to this is that norms are counterfactually valid – their existence is not necessarily refuted by instances of noncompliance. Friedrich Kratochwil and John Ruggie draw a useful comparison with domestic laws on drunk driving, asking

> Does driving while under the influence of alcohol refute the law (norm) against drunk driving? Does it when half the population is implicated? To be sure, the law (norm) is *violated* thereby. But whether or not violations also invalidate or refute a law (norm) will depend upon a host of other factors, not the least of which is how the community assesses the violation and responds to it. (1986: 767; emphasis in original)

Where a justification for non-compliance is not offered, or where the one offered is seen as inadequate, we commonly see other members of international society criticising the behaviour of the noncompliant state. The presence or absence of condemnation in cases of noncompliance, therefore, becomes a useful test of the strength of a norm – an issue to which we return in our discussion of the influenza case study.

The reason we adopt this ideationally-oriented constructivist approach is that we believe that the changes we have seen in the global disease control regime in recent years can best be understood as the product of significant changes in shared understandings about disease, security, and sovereignty. Our intention in this chapter therefore has been to evaluate recent events using a constructivist lens to test those assumptions, rather than revisiting ongoing debates that compare constructivism against alternative rationalist or realist approaches. In particular, while material changes to the global environment (for example, increased cross-border travel and trade) were partly responsible for motivating the IHR revisions – and indeed the IHR revisions have often been portrayed as a rational response to a heightened threat – we can only appreciate why states have agreed to such onerous demands and limitations on their sovereignty by taking into account some important ideational changes that have taken place. In particular, the 'securitization' of disease, which has broadened understandings of what constitutes a 'global security threat', has fundamentally changed the previously predominant view that how states manage health crises is primarily a domestic concern. The revised IHR were a product of this changed understanding, and have in turn acted as an engine of socialization, requiring states to adopt certain structures, practices and behaviours in the name of advancing collective 'global health security'. Why states agreed to impose common standards on things such as surveillance infrastructure requirements and verification timeframes, despite the vast health inequalities amongst states and the huge differences in their domestic health systems, and why they agreed to the limitations on their freedom to impose health measures, can only be appreciated when the power of the social construct behind the global health security idea is understood (Davies et al. forthcoming).

Whether international norms *matter* (in other words, whether they affect state behaviour) has been a long-running debate in International Relations theory. Some of the more sophisticated realist theorists do accept that a norm-driven 'logic of appropriateness' influences state behaviour in some circumstances (Krasner 1999); although they would not expect states to comply where they didn't see that compliance as being in their interests. Alternatively, theorists in the neoliberal institutionalist mould would see norms such as the IHR provisions on additional health measures as examples of rational cooperative action, a result of their contention that states in such circumstances prefer cooperation (and the absolute gains it brings) over competition and an obsession with relative gains, as realists claim (Keohane 1984). In other words, institutionalists would see cooperation and coordination through the IHR as the product of a rational response to interdependency.[1]

Yet crucial to the constructivist case is the idea that states are not engaged in a constant process of calculating how to maximise their interests, but rather that compliance is 'a matter of applying socially generated convictions and understandings about how national interests are likely to be achieved in any particular policy domain' (Haas 2000: 62). The constructivist approach adopted here is fundamentally different from rational choice theories in how it understands the ways in which those interests (and indeed the identities of actors) are formed, and in particular the extent to which they are 'at stake' in social interactions. Rational

---

1   For a comparison of realist, neoliberal and 'cognitivist' approaches to international regimes see Hasenclever et al. (1997: 1–7).

choice theories tend to view actors' identities and interests as exogenously given, and where they do change this is likely to be a consequence of material changes. The constructivist approach, on the other hand, views identities and interests as 'constituted' through social interactions. According to this view, the identities and interests of states are inevitably affected by their participation in the international system, and therefore by prevailing international norms. States internalize norms, and for the most part tend to understand their interests, and therefore behave, in accordance with those norms in an almost 'subconscious' fashion. Thus, approaches that treat interests as exogenously given and identities as essentially stable fail to account for some of the more interesting ways in which the global response to cross-border disease threats has changed.

These different theoretical approaches translate into very different expectations about compliance. Such is the challenge to state sovereignty posed by the new provisions on additional health measures that realists would expect relatively low levels of compliance. Realists, of course, would only consider compliance likely if a state deemed that to be in its interests in any case, or if the rule was backed by some kind of enforcement capability (for example, if the rules are enforced by a global hegemon). In the case of IHR (2005), as we mentioned above, no such enforcement mechanism exists. Neoliberal institutionalist scholars, by contrast, have made the case that realists tend to underestimate the degree of compliance that we see in practice. They have explained this via an emphasis on the incentives that states have in long-term stable cooperation – even in some cases at the expense of some short-term costs– and on the ways in which institutions can be designed in ways to reduce the likelihood of non-compliance.

Yet these explanations both rest on the assumption that states' understandings of their interests remain essentially static and that they act as rational utility-maximizers. Whilst, to reiterate, we are not engaged here in testing these explanations against each other, we argue that the process leading up to the IHR revisions, and subsequent events, do seem to have changed underlying assumptions about the roles and interests of international actors. When states agreed to the revised IHR framework they subscribed to new expectations of each other, new material requirements and new social norms. States are role players in the global health security regime and, as we will see below, tend to play (and expect others to properly play) their roles. If the constructivists' explanation for norm-compliance is to be plausible then we would expect to see certain things happen in cases of noncompliance with a norm which is widely seen as a legitimate behavioural expectation. In simplified form, social constructivists would expect that:

- Most states will comply most of the time;
- Compliance would not be a conscious calculation but rather that states form their understanding of their interests in the light of the norm;
- Compliance may well become routinized, for example in bureaucratic procedures and processes;

- Instances of non-compliance (which are possible) will be accompanied by attempts by the non-compliant state to justify its behaviour;
- Noncompliance will be criticized by other states, even if they do not usually go so far as to take enforcement action; and
- Such criticisms will be couched in terms of the norm: that the non-compliant state has failed to live up to the behavioural expectations of its peers.

In the next section we investigate compliance with the IHR's additional health measures rules in the case of the 2009 H1N1 influenza pandemic as a 'plausibility probe' in order to examine the extent to which these constructivist expectations have been met. Of particular interest is whether or not there is evidence in that discourse to support a constructivist reading of the new regulations, and if so what the history of the H1N1 pandemic can tell us about the current state of compliance and internalization.

The 2009 H1N1 Influenza Pandemic and IHR Compliance

Particularly since 2005, the international community has invested considerable human, financial, and technical resources in preparing for another influenza pandemic. For many, the 2003 SARS outbreak was considered a 'wake-up call', demonstrating just how rapidly communicable diseases could spread around the world and the economic damage that such events could inflict, even when large numbers of human fatalities did not occur (Basur et al. 2004: 22). The subsequent emergence and progressive global dissemination of the H5N1 influenza virus (commonly referred to as 'Bird Flu', also see Chapter 8) from late 2003 onwards reinforced the message that another pandemic remained a distinct probability. In the view of many public health officials, it was not a matter of 'if' but 'when'. In November 2005, just six months after IHR (2005) had been endorsed by the 58th WHA, the international community met again at the WHO headquarters in Geneva, Switzerland, to develop a strategy to strengthen global pandemic preparedness. According to the joint United Nations System Influenza Coordinator (UNSIC) and World Bank's 2010 report, between 2005 and 2009 some US$4.3 billion was allocated to strengthening public health response efforts, enhancing disease surveillance capabilities, and boosting global production capacity for developing influenza vaccines and antiviral medications (UNSIC and World Bank 2010: 31).

In April 2009, this investment appeared to be both timely and appropriate following the revelation that a novel strain of H1N1 influenza had the previous month in La Gloria, Mexico, successfully achieved human-to-human transmission. However, due to Mexico's limited laboratory capacity, it took some weeks before the US Centers for Disease Control and Prevention and Canadian health authorities were able to confirm on 23 April that a novel strain had indeed emerged, by which time the virus had already spread internationally (Cohen 2009). WHO published its first global alert regarding the outbreak the next day, 24 April 2009 (WHO 2009a).

Following the global alert, WHO urged the international community to launch an aggressive and widespread public health campaign to combat the H1N1 threat. Due to the fact that the outbreak was caused by a novel strain of influenza, Director-General Margaret Chan invoked the IHR (2005) for the first time and convened the inaugural meeting of IHR Emergency Committee on 25 April 2009, drawing together scientific experts to provide technical advice and recommendations on what measures should be taken. On the basis of this Committee's advice, on 27 April 2009 the alert status was raised from Phase 3 (limited transmission) to Phase 4 (community-level outbreaks) (WHO 2009c), and eventually, on 11 June 2009, to Phase 6 (Pandemic) (WHO 2009g). The WHO Secretariat also began to issue daily (and in some instances twice-daily) updates on the global situation, as well as to publish various recommendations and technical advice on such matters as surveillance and monitoring, the safety and efficacy of vaccines, and measures aimed at reducing exposure to the virus (WHO 2009f).

In an attempt to circumvent the risk that the outbreak would become known as the 'Mexican Flu' (and the inevitable economic damage that would result to Mexico if such an association developed) the WHO initially labelled the outbreak 'Swine Flu' on account of the fact that the H1N1 virus was also found to infect pigs. Within days, however, it became apparent that some countries were employing additional health measures that seemed to contravene the object and purpose of the IHR (2005). These included:

- Egyptian authorities in late April ordering the mass culling of all pigs throughout the country (estimated between 250,000 to 400,000 livestock), even though there had been no recorded cases of human H1N1 in the country, nor any reported outbreaks of H1N1 in pigs worldwide;
- Government authorities in China and Singapore beginning to automatically quarantine tourists (notably Mexican, American, and Canadian citizens) based on their nationality or because they had recently travelled to Mexico, irrespective of their potential exposure to the virus;
- Several countries – including Argentina, Cuba, Ecuador, and Peru – issuing immediate temporary suspension orders on all flights to Mexico, and to North America generally;
- More than 20 countries imposing import bans on live pigs, pork and pork products, citing concerns over the risk of H1N1 infection (Katz and Fischer 2010; Hodge 2010).

All these actions went far beyond the measures suggested by the WHO, which had issued a statement as early as 26 April 2009 that trade and travel restrictions were not recommended (WHO 2009b). On 27 April 2009, the Secretariat expanded on its advice, explicitly stating 'There is also no risk of infection from this virus from consumption of well-cooked pork and pork products' (WHO 2009e). On 30 April 2009, the Food and Agriculture Organization (FAO), World Organization for Animal

Health (OIE) and WHO then issued a joint statement (re-issued on 7 May 2009) stipulating that pork and pork products were safe (WHO 2009d). Nonetheless, a small number of countries persisted with travel restrictions and/or live pig and pork import bans to the extent that in late June 2009 a series of complaints were formally lodged with WTO (WTO 2009h). These restrictions, which directly contravened WHO advice, were prima facie breaches of the additional health measures norm. The responses to those cases of non-compliance, and the justification put forward in support of them, are examined in the remainder of this section.

Those countries most affected by the pork import bans and travel restrictions (notably, Mexico, the United States, and Canada) were understandably quick to condemn them. Canada's trade minister, for example, openly rebuked the governments responsible. Invoking the principles outlined in the IHR (2005) that additional health measures needed to substantiated by sound scientific evidence, the minister observed that governments should 'make decisions that are scientifically based ... We would expect those countries, which have gone ahead with the ban or were thinking about it, would stop and have a look at scientific guidelines and would recognise that the meat itself is not a problem' (MacInnis 2009). Likewise, China's actions in, firstly, quarantining Mexican citizens without just cause, and then later imposing pork bans, received a strong admonition from the Mexican authorities and prompted WHO to formally request the public health rationale for China's actions under the IHR (2005) (Fidler 2009).

Such arguments from the 'victims' of travel and trade restrictions are perhaps to be expected but, adding weight to the suggestion that the norm on additional health measures was widely seen as valid, even those countries that were not large pork exporters or that did not have citizens forcibly quarantined, joined with affected countries in the context of the WTO in condemning the trade and travel restrictions, criticizing those governments who imposed them while praising those countries who based their decisions on science. Although the WHO Secretariat refrained from 'naming and shaming' those countries that contravened IHR (2005), other United Nations agencies were not so restrained. A representative of FAO roundly condemned the actions of the Egyptian authorities, labelling the slaughter of the indigenous pig population as 'a real mistake' (Stewart 2009).

Indeed, even though only a small proportion of countries – approximately 10% of WHO's 194 member states – knowingly contravened the IHR (reflecting the idea that most countries comply most of the time), it is also clear that many of those states that did not comply knew their actions required at least some form of justification, indicating that they recognised to some extent the validity of the norm regarding additional health measures. However, interestingly, non-compliant states' justifications for their behaviour were not always the evidence-based public health rationales required under IHR (2005); instead, in some cases, they argued why they thought that breaching the norm was justifiable in the prevailing circumstances. Countries such as Iraq, for example, which had slaughtered three wild boars in a Baghdad zoo, admitted that its actions were not based on science but rather were intended 'to break a barrier of fear' amongst zoo visitors (Karadesh

2009). Similarly the Philippines – which had banned pork imports from the United States, Mexico, and Canada on 25 April 2009 as a 'precautionary measure' (Joshi 2009) – lifted the ban less than a week later for the US and Mexico and maintained the ban on Canada only because there was reportedly a suspected case of swine-to-human H1N1 (Ager 2009). In other cases, states went so far as to apologise for their non-compliance. As early as 4 May 2009, for example, the Chinese authorities released a statement that they were not intentionally discriminating against Mexican citizens (BBC 2009). The following month the Chinese health minister formally apologised to his Mexican counterpart, expressing regret for not discussing his country's containment strategy earlier and praising the Mexican government for its transparency throughout the pandemic (AFP 2009). Later, when confronted in WTO, China again sought to justify its actions on the basis of 'its large vulnerable population, the burden on its public health system, the importance of pigs and pork, and the fact that the H1N1 virus shares some genetic make-up with influenza that affects pigs' (WTO 2009h).

Admittedly, a smaller subset of governments remained staunchly unapologetic, even antagonistic, to the suggestion that their actions were irresponsible. Arguably the most extreme illustration of this was demonstrated by Russia's chief veterinary officer, Nikolai Vlasov, when he stated he not only agreed with Russia's ban on pork imports, but that 'Health officials should stick to their own business and not promote the world pork trade' (Budrys 2009). Elsewhere, a small number of countries such as Indonesia, Egypt, Ukraine, North Korea, and Ghana simply failed to provide any justification or explanation for their actions whatsoever. Taking note of the fact that many of the countries that had imposed the pork import bans are comprised of predominantly Muslim populations, speculation understandably emerged that the bans were religiously motivated (Audi 2009). Certainly, the silence demonstrated by these countries would seem to indicate that the process of socialization around the additional health measures norm is not yet fully complete, as – at least according to a constructivist reading – it would be reasonable to expect that most if not all countries that contravened the norm would seek to explain their actions to some degree. The lack of any attempt by these states to justify the additional health measures thereby suggests only two possible explanations: (a) they simply viewed the international community's condemnation with little regard, suggesting they placed little or no value in IHR (2005)'s norms; or (b) they recognized there was no reasonable justification for their actions, and so silence was used as a strategy to avoid international attention and thereby minimize any further condemnation and/ or repercussions. Given that IHR (2005)'s framework was passed with unanimous approval in May 2005 (Wilson et al. 2008), and that WHO's global health security function has been further endorsed and reinforced in May 2011 (WHO 2011), we maintain that the latter of these two explanations is the more likely in most cases; although some states – North Korea being the most obvious example – habitually show little concern for international condemnation of their actions.

It is again important to note, however, that the majority of countries fully complied with the IHR norm regarding additional health measures. For the most part, WHO recommendations were strictly adhered to, and governments were quick to indicate where their actions were based on sound scientific evidence and where uncertainty remained (Fogarty et al. 2011). Adding weight to the case that the majority of countries had internalized the norm, governments were also observed giving their respective domestic populations very little justification for why they were not implementing more severe trade and travel restrictions to prevent the further importation of the H1N1 virus. Instead, the overwhelming focus was on how countries could help reduce illness via vaccination or the use of antiviral medications, combined with measures that individuals could take to mitigate their personal risk of contracting influenza.

Conclusion

The 2009 H1N1 pandemic represented the first invocation of the revised IHR, and the first opportunity to judge the extent to which states had internalized the new norms surrounding additional health measures. Overall there seems to be evidence to suggest that the majority of the international community have internalized the revised IHR (2005) additional health measures norm. As we have observed above, the vast majority of countries did comply, refraining from imposing restrictions in excess of the WHO Director-General's recommendations even though domestically it may have been politically expedient to implement tougher restrictions. Thus, even though there was significant noncompliance (in that approximately 10 per cent of countries applied measures that contravened the additional health measures norm) most states did in fact comply.

Moreover, there is sufficient evidence to suggest that the majority of states complied with the IHR norm regarding additional health measures not from a sense of obligation per se, but rather because they had internalized the principle it represents. Put another way, even though the decision to comply with the IHR may have represented a rational choice for some countries, based either on a sense of legal obligation or short-term policy objectives, it can also be reasonably argued that governments complied with IHR (2005) because they had actually come to believe that the norms enshrined within the framework reflect a preferred system for interstate cooperation. As the next chapter will demonstrate, when IHR (2005) are viewed historically, governments have substantially redefined their interests. Seen in this light, compliance with the IHR in the context of the 2009 H1N1 influenza pandemic reflects a more profound, deep-seated change in states' perceptions of their interests (for a dissenting view, see Chapter 8); and we could reasonably expect to see compliance in the future become routinized, reflected, for instance, in bureaucratic procedures and processes, and codified in national law (the details of which are further discussed in Chapter 10).

Of those countries that failed to comply, at least half sought to justify their actions for doing so and, along with those countries that remained silent, all were openly criticized and publicly rebuked over their breach of protocol. It seems, then, that most of the expectations of constructivist scholars were indeed borne out in the case examined here, and that states have willingly traded elements of state sovereignty to ensure greater health security. Nevertheless, it has to be admitted that there was a relatively high level of noncompliance in the first real test of IHR (2005). Realist scholars would no doubt seize on this as evidence that their predictions are correct and that what occurred throughout the H1N1 pandemic was proof that states happily ignore international law when it does not coincide with their interests, at least if there is little prospect of noncompliance leading to enforcement action. We contend, however, that a better explanation is that the norm socialization and internalization process is currently incomplete – not surprising given that the norms embodied within IHR (2005) are new. Moreover, the technological changes underway in surveillance, as chapters 5 and 6 will illustrate, test even the most recalcitrant reporting state to keep news of an outbreak quiet. It is clearly problematic to draw too many bold conclusions on the basis of a single case. Given that new communicable diseases and other public health risks are continuing to emerge at an alarming rate, however, there is little doubt that compliance with the 'additional health measures' norm will soon be tested again.

Acknowledgements

Work on this chapter was funded by the European Research Council under the European Community's Seventh Framework Programme – Ideas Grant 230489 GHG.

References

Ager, M. 2009. Import Ban on Pork Lifted, Except Canada. *Inquirer.net* [Online, 4 May] Available at: http://newsinfo.inquirer.net/breakingnews/nation/view/20090504-203022/Import-ban-on-pork-lifted-except-Canada [Accessed: 14 July 2011].

Associated French Press. China Apologises to Mexico for Tough H1N1 Flu Stand. *Channelnewsasia.com* [Online, 4 July] Available at: http://www.channelnewsasia.com/stories/afp_asiapacific/view/440320/1/.html [Accessed: 14 July 2011].

Audi, N. 2009. Culling Pigs in Flu Fight, Egypt Angers Herders and Dismays U.N. *New York Times* [Online, 30 April] Available at: http://www.nytimes.com/2009/05/01/health/01egypt.html [Accessed: 14 July 2011].

Basrur, S.V., Yaffe, B. and Henry, B. 2004. SARS: A Local Public Health Perspective. *Canadian Journal of Public Health*, 95 (1), 22–4.

BBC. China Denies Flu Discrimination. *BBC World Service* [Online, 4 May] Available at: http://news.bbc.co.uk/1/hi/world/asia-pacific/8032157.stm [Accessed: 14 July 2011].

Budrys, A. 2009. Russia Says Extend Pork Import Ban to Canada, Spain. *Reuters* [Online, 4 May] Available at: http://www.reuters.com/article/2009/05/04/us-flu-russia-idUSTRE5431PB20090504 [Accessed: 14 July 2011].

Cash, R.A. and Narasimhan, V. 2000. Impediments to Global Surveillance of Infectious Diseases: Consequences of Open Reporting in a Global Economy. *Bulletin of the World Health Organisation*, 78 (11), 1358–67.

Cohen, J. 2009. Out of Mexico? Scientists Ponder Swine Flu's Origins. *Science*, 324 (5928), 700–702.

Davies, S., Kamradt-Scott, A. and Rushton, S. (forthcoming). *Disease Diplomacy: Politics, Pandemics and Global Health Security*. Baltimore, MA: Johns Hopkins University Press.

Fidler, D.P. 2005. From International Sanitary Conventions to Global Health Security: The New International Health Regulations. *Chinese Journal of International Law*, 4 (2), 325–92.

____. 2009. H1N1 After Action Review: Learning from the Unexpected, the Success and the Fear. *Future Microbiology*, 4 (7), 767–9.

Finnemore, M. 2000. Are Legal Norms Distinctive? *International Law and Politics*, 3 (3), 699–705.

Fogarty, A.S., Holland, K., Imison, M., et al. 2011. Communicating Uncertainty – How Australian Television Reported H1N1 Risk in 2009: A Content Analysis. *BMC Public Health*, 11 (1), 181–9.

Haas, P.M. 2000. Choosing to Comply: Theorizing from International Relations and Comparative Politics, in *Commitment and Compliance: The Role of Non-binding Norms in the International Legal System*, edited by D. Shelton. Oxford: Oxford University Press, 43–64.

Hasenclever, A., Mayer, P. and Rittberger, V. 1997. *Theories of International Regimes*. Cambridge: Cambridge University Press.

Hodge, J.G. 2010. Global Legal Triage in Response to the 2009 H1N1 Outbreak. *Minnesota Journal of Law, Science & Technology*, 11 (2), 599–628.

Joshi, M. 2009. Philippines Bans Pork Imports from Mexico, US. *TopNews* [Online, 25 April] Available at: http://www.topnews.in/philippines-bans-pork-imports-mexico-us-2156861 [Accessed: 14 September 2011].

Kamradt-Scott, A. 2010. The WHO Secretariat, Norm Entrepreneurship, and Global Disease Outbreak Control. *Journal of International Organizations Studies*, 1 (1), 72–89.

Karadesh, J. 2009. Wild Boars killed in Iraq over Swine Flu Fears. *CNN.com* [Online, 3 May] Available at: http://edition.cnn.com/2009/WORLD/meast/05/03/iraq.boars/ [Accessed: 14 July 2011].

Katz, R. and Fischer, J. 2010. The Revised International Health Regulations: A Framework for Global Pandemic Response. *Global Health Governance*, 3 (2), 1–18.

Keohane, R. 1984. *After Hegemony: Cooperation and Discord in the World Political Economy*. Princeton, NJ: Princeton University Press.

Krasner, S.D. 1999. *Sovereignty: Organized Hypocrisy*. Princeton, NJ: Princeton University Press.

Kratchowil, F. and Ruggie, J.G. 1986. International Organization: A State of the Art on the Art of the State. *International Organization*, 40 (4), 753–75.

MacInnis, L. 2009. Mexico Says Pork Import Bans Unjustified, Illegal. *Reuters* [Online, 5 May] Available at: http://uk.reuters.com/article/2009/05/05/idUKL5956461 [Accessed: 14 July 2011].

Neff, S.C. 2002. A Short History of International Law, in *International Law*, edited by M.E. Evans. Oxford: Oxford University Press, 31–58.

Stewart, P. 2009. UN Agency Slams Egypt Order to Cull All Pigs. *Reuters* [Online, 29 April] Available at: http://www.reuters.com/article/2009/04/29/idUSLT11250 [Accessed: 14 July 2011].

United Nations System Influenza Coordinator, and World Bank 2010. *Animal and Pandemic Influenza: A Framework for Sustaining Momentum*. Bangkok: UNSIC and World Bank.

van Tigerstrom, B. 2006. The Revised International Health Regulations and Restraint on National Health Measures. *Health Law Journal*, 13, 35–76.

Wendt, A. 1992. Anarchy is What States Make of It: The Social Construction of Power Politics. *International Organization*, 46 (2), 391–425.

Wilson, K., McDougall, C., Fidler, D.P. and Lazar, H. 2008. Strategies for Implementing the New International Health Regulations in Federal Countries. *Bulletin of the World Health Organization*, 86 (3), 215–20.

World Health Organization 1951. *International Sanitary Regulations*. Geneva: WHO Press.

____. 1969. *International Health Regulations (1969)*. Geneva: WHO Press.

____. 2005. *International Health Regulations (2005)*. Geneva: WHO Press.

____. 2009a. *Influenza-like Illness in the United States and Mexico. Global Alert and Response (GAR), 24 April 2009*. [Online]. Available at: http://www.who.int/csr/don/2009_04_24/en/index.html [Accessed: 14 July 2011].

____. 2009b. *Swine Flu Illness in the United States and Mexico – Update 2. Global Alert and Response (GAR)*. [Online]. Available at: http://www.who.int/csr/don/2009_04_26/en/index.html [Accessed: 15 July 2011].

____. 2009c. *Swine Influenza – Statement by WHO Director-General, Dr Margaret Chan. Media Centre, 27 April 2009*. [Online]. Available at: http://www.who.int/mediacentre/news/statements/2009/h1n1_20090427/en/ [Accessed: 14 July 2011].

____. 2009d. *Joint FAO/WHO/OIE Statement on Influenza A(H1N1) and the Safety of Pork. WHO Media Centre – Statements*. [Online]. Available at: http://www.who.int/mediacentre/news/statements/2009/h1n1_20090430/en/index.html [Accessed: 14 July 2011].

____. 2009e. *Swine Influenza – Update 3. Global Alert and Response (GAR)*. [Online]. Available at: http://www.who.int/csr/don/2009_04_27/en/index.html [Accessed: 13 July 2011].

____. 2009f. *Pandemic Influenza Prevention and Mitigation in Low Resource Communities*. [Online]. Available at: http://www.who.int/csr/resources/publica

tions/swineflu/PI_summary_low_resource_02_05_2009.pdf [Accessed: 15 July 2011].

____. 2009g. *DG Statement Following the Meeting of the Emergency Committee. Global Alert and Response (GAR), 11 June 2009.* [Online]. Available at: http://www.who.int/csr/disease/swineflu/4th_meeting_ihr/en/ [accessed 14 July 2011].

____. 2009h. *Members Discuss Trade Responses to H1N1 Flu. World Trade Organization Sanitary and Phytosanitary Measures.* [Online]. Available at: http://www.wto.org/english/news_e/news09_e/sps_25jun09_e.htm [accessed 14 July 2011].

____. 2011. *WHO Reform: World Health Assembly Resolution WHA64.2.* [Online]. Available at: http://apps.who.int/gb/ebwha/pdf_files/WHA64/A64_R2-en.pdf [accessed 15 July 2011].

Chapter 3

Risk Perception, Assessment, and Management in Responses to Pandemic Influenza

Theresa Seetoh, Marco Liverani, and Richard Coker

Introduction

Three influenza pandemics occurred during the twentieth century. The 1918 'Spanish influenza' was noted for its exceptional virulence (Cunha 2004), killing an estimated 50 million people (Centers for Disease Control 2011) while the 1957 'Asian Influenza' and the 1968 'Hong Kong influenza' saw the emergence of novel viral strains (Palese 2004). In the past few years, concerns about the public health and economic impact of new pandemic threats have increased. In 2005, David Nabarro, the United Nations coordinator for avian and human influenza, announced that a pandemic of avian influenza could kill up to 150 million people worldwide (BBC 2005). More recently, the World Bank (2008) estimated that an influenza pandemic would cost the world US$3 trillion, and would shrink the global economy by up to 4.8%.

As a result of these growing concerns, governments have made huge investments in pandemic influenza preparedness and control, with worldwide expenditures more than tripling from US$2.2 billion in 2004 to US$7 billion in 2009 (Market Research Media 2011). Dr Margaret Chan, Director-General of the World Health Organization (WHO), noted that 'investing in pandemic preparedness is essentially like investing in an insurance policy' (Chan 2006). The unpredictable nature of an influenza pandemic, and its potential consequences on society, raises the important question of whether public health professionals across various contexts can assess and interpret the pandemic risk accurately and consistently and, if not, manage uncertainty in a competent manner.

The focus on surveillance in this chapter is to explore how it informs risk perception, assessment, and management in the community. As such, the first section in this chapter explores what is 'risk' and how is it framed[1] in the practice of pandemic influenza policy and control? To examine this question, we reviewed the

1   In this study, we take the word 'frame' to mean how public health policies are determined by its actors, context, content, decision-making processes and the interrelations among these factors (Walt and Gilson 1994).

literature on the assessment, perception and management of risk in two episodes of influenza with pandemic potential: the 1976 swine flu scare in the USA and the 2004 H5N1 avian influenza emergency in Thailand, as well as the 2009 H1N1 pandemic influenza. From these cases we develop a conceptual abstraction which we detail in the final section of the chapter in order to illustrate the dynamics driving public health policy in these three historical cases. We suggest policy-makers are, for the most part, unaware that their surveillance and risk modelling tools presently narrow the range of risk management decisions that may be required to facilitate outbreak control.

Methods

Our literature search was conducted from June to August 2011 on a variety of sources (Patton 2002), including scientific and grey literature,[2] as well as media reports by established news agencies. The analysis of risk in pandemic influenza policy and control required two separate literature reviews: one on methodological and practical problems in risk analysis, and another on the practice of risk management as it pertains to pandemic influenza policy and control. The literature search was conducted using JSTOR and PubMed as databases. Specific details on the literature search can be found in an article we have previously published on this research (Seetoh et al. 2012). Qualitative analysis was performed iteratively alongside data collection.[3] Reliability and validity concerns (Aveyard 2007; Golafshani 2003) were addressed by using a structured search strategy (such as the consistent use of search terms and selection criteria) and cross-referencing sources for mutual reinforcement (Lincoln and Guba 1985). Finally, based on the above review, we developed a conceptual framework that sheds light on the relationships between risk assessment, risk perception and risk management identified as the three main elements driving the making of public health policy in these case studies.[4]

---

2   Examples of grey literature include technical reports and articles from governments and international organizations, and working papers from research groups.

3   A quantitative presentation of the literature reviewed, such as a systematic meta-analysis, could have been useful if the research involved a numerical synthesis of statistical risk estimates. However, for the purpose of this research, which involves the development of a conceptual abstraction on risk based on the concept and practice of risk in pandemic influenza policy, quantitative analysis is inadequate and inappropriate in capturing the rich conceptual explanations on risk. A qualitative analysis, on the other hand, aids the reviewer in elucidating and contextualizing the concept of risk (Green and Thorogood 2004; Patton 2002) with inference to recurring themes (Cooper 1982) based on the information reviewed.

4   Reliability, applicability and parsimony were considered in the design of the conceptual framework. Reliability involves the use of multiple sources to cross-reference evidence (Patton 2002), such as the consultation of a variety of sources in the decision to include specific components in the conceptual framework. Applicability refers to how

Results – A Brief Overview of 'risk'

In probabilistic terms, 'risk' can be expressed as the likelihood of an event occurring given a set of initial conditions and parameters affecting outcomes (Crouchy et al. 2006; Menon 2011). In the context of public health, risk assessment typically involves the quantification of risk factors using a risk matrix, defined by a vertical axis of relative impact and a horizontal axis of relative likelihood. The risk of an event is then calculated by multiplying the consequences of the event against the probability of event occurrence (UK Health Protection Agency 2011):

Risk = ¼ consequences of the event x probability of event occurrence.

Real-life complexity, however, escapes neat estimations by probabilistic methods alone. Scientists concede the inability of mechanistic models to fully capture aspects of population heterogeneity, behavioural change and other social phenomena (Timpka et al. 2009). Such incapacity can significantly undermine the predictive power of risk modelling, especially in situations where population behaviour is disrupted by the catastrophic consequences of a high-impact event (Ferguson 2007). Furthermore, the genetic variation in pathogens complicates responses. Even if scientists are able to identify a new virus, they cannot necessarily preview or predict how that virus will actually interact within the human population.

Adding to this complexity, current risk assessment techniques are further challenged by issues resulting from its relationship with risk management. The boundary between risk assessment and risk management lacks clear distinction, as these two elements cannot operate in isolation from one another (Gerrard and Petts 1998; US EPA 2011). Risk managers require evidence-based inputs, while risk analysis is subjected to validation by risk managers (Rip 1986; Tierney 1999). In addition, risk management is not based on the outcomes of risk assessment alone, but is influenced by a range of other factors, including the institutional and public health contexts in which decisions are made (Jasanoff 1993; Moore 1977; Renn and Rohrmann 2000). For example, risk management capacity (that is, the availability of control options in the event of an influenza pandemic) may influence the decision to adopt either a containment or mitigation strategy. The proven benefits of an available risk management option may further perceptually overestimate the need to react to a potential risk (Atun and Gurol-Urganci 2005; Jasanoff 1993; Moore 1977; Renn and Rohrmann 2000).

In sum, improved understanding of risk ought to account for the complexity of interactions between the different components that coincide to produce

---

widely the conceptual framework can be generalized, and this leads to the development of a framework based on broad but applicable factors. Parsimony involves limiting the components essential for the framework on risk such that the number of components in the framework is kept sufficiently small.

policy decisions through the interplay between risk assessment, risk perception and risk management.

Demarcating Risk Assessment and Risk Management:
The 1976 Swine Influenza 'Pandemic'

Following cases of influenza among new recruits at Fort Dix in New Jersey in 1976, scientists at the US Centers for Disease Control and Prevention (CDC) deemed the chance of an influenza pandemic occurring as 'probable'. Risk assessment was based on the likelihood of cases to have had human-to-human transmission and the observed phenomenon that a human pandemic almost always follows an antigenic shift in the current circulating virus. This assessment was further supported by the perception that a human influenza pandemic was long overdue. On the risk management end, both scientists and politicians had access to an influenza vaccine containing the swine influenza strain (Fineberg and Neustadt 1978), although concerns were raised over its potential side-effects. Reservations notwithstanding, US President Gerald Ford ordered the mass immunization of the American population. The 'pandemic scare' itself eventually resulted in an outbreak that killed only one person and hospitalized 13, while adverse reactions to the vaccine caused thousands of cases of Guillain–Barré syndrome and 25 deaths.

Many analysts argued that the management of the 1976 influenza was a political and public health fiasco (Beck 2009; Durodie 2004, Menon 2008; Siegel 2006). Further, some reviewers argued that the interference of politics in science, along with the proactive engagement of scientists in the process of policy-making, compromised the autonomy and judgement of the two categories of stakeholders (Beck 2009; Fineberg and Neustadt 1978). Critical studies of risk have demonstrated that it is not possible for risk assessment to remain value-free in the midst of its close linkages with risk management processes, such as policy-making (Adams 1995, Mansnerus 2010; Tesh 1988; Tierney 1999). Moreover, risk assessment is often shrouded in epistemic uncertainties (Freudenburg 1996; Porter 1995), and the inability of scientists to accurately predict the timing and impact of the next emerging pandemic bears witness to the limitations of prospective knowledge in pandemic preparedness (Menon 2008). Walter Dowdle (1997), a virologist at the US CDC, recalled in an interview:

> It was clear we could not say the virus would spread. But it was clear that there had been human-to-human spread […] We had to report our fundamental belief that a pandemic was indeed a possibility. (Fineberg and Neustadt 1978)

Such high uncertainty contexts may drive risk managers to overlook public health considerations in favour of political interests. In 1976, the pandemic emergency coinciding with the presidential primaries contributed to the adoption of an interventionist approach, as the catastrophic impact of a pandemic could have marred President Ford's re-election campaign. In a subsequent interview, Ford said he would 'rather gamble on the side of caution and be ahead of the curve than behind it' (Fineberg and Neustadt 1978). Thus, the adoption of a strong precautionary approach was justified from a political standpoint despite the absence of strong scientific evidence.

Contextualizing Avian Influenza: Local and Global Political Economy Concerns

From 2004 to 2008, the avian influenza virus infected a total of 25 persons in Thailand, with 17 confirmed deaths (Chompook et al. 2009). Globally, 396 human cases were reported from December 2003 to April 2006, with an overall case fatality ratio of 60% (WHO 2008). As a result of this emergency, Thai Premier Thaksin Shinawatra ordered the mass culling of 40 million chickens and fowls between January and April 2004 (Bloomberg 2004). Japan and the European Union, two of Thailand's largest poultry export markets, reacted to the outbreak by banning imports of frozen chicken from the country. In the wake of these developments, Shinawatra tried to play down the pandemic risk and threatened 'trade retaliation' against countries that banned its exports. He went further by staging a public appearance where he was seen 'cheerfully tucking into a variety of spicy Thai chicken dishes' (Perrin 2004) and mobilized all Thais to 'unite and eat chicken' in order to secure the nation's economic interests (The Nation 2004a). The skilful diversion of the avian influenza outbreak (The Nation 2004b) from a public health concern to its implications for the Thai economy is a prominent example of how risk assessment can be framed strategically to inform risk perception. In Thailand, the avian influenza risk was largely shaped by the economic imperatives of the poultry industry. The country was the world's fourth largest poultry exporter (Nicita 2007), and estimates suggested that the poultry industry provided more than 400,000 jobs nationwide (Tiensin et al. 2005). The country's avian influenza epidemic, couples with the subsequent ban of Thai exports by its trading partners, brought significant adverse economic repercussions. At the peak of the epidemic, Thai poultry exports were estimated to have fallen from US$500 million in 2002 to almost zero in 2005 (Nicita 2007). The Charoen Pokphand (CP) Group, Thailand's largest poultry conglomerate, was the hardest hit. Given the pivotal role of the poultry industry in the Thai economy and the influence of livestock entrepreneurs on the government, government officials felt compelled to protect and bail the industry from the epidemic's impact (Safman 2009). At the same time, frontline workers, such as doctors and the military, were not adequately informed of the actual extent of the epidemic (Tangwisutijit 2005), and this produced negative effects on containment and mitigation efforts.

The centrality of Thailand in the Southeast Asian region and its intense trade relations with member countries in the Association of Southeast Asian Nations

(ASEAN) and the Asia-Pacific Economic Cooperation (APEC) forum also contributed to the framing of pandemic risk in economic terms, albeit for different reasons. During the APEC summit in 2005, the risk of avian influenza turning pandemic was addressed as one of the most important regional issues (Olsen and Harvey 2005), given the rapid spread of the disease across national borders and the high level of human mobility throughout the region.

In connection with the advent of surveillance technology, there has been a shift of risk perception from a national to an international dimension that is an increasingly important element in shaping public health policy (Mintz and Redd 2003). As Chapter 1 highlighted, since the International Sanitary Conventions in the nineteenth century, it has become apparent that the transnational spread of diseases cannot merely be a matter of national governance but is one that requires standard procedures, international communication channels and common agreements on the handling of infected travellers across borders (Howard-Jones 1975, Fidler 2005). However, the international dimension of communicable disease policy has increasingly been driven by a realist agenda, perpetuating a global outbreak narrative that can reinforce the perception of risk in terms of economic and security costs (Scoones and Forster 2010). This view has been propagated by the International Health Regulations, a document that, in all its subsequent revisions, has emphasized the importance of minimizing any undue interference in international commerce by adopting intervention measures commensurate with the public health risk involved (for more discussion of the revisions prior to adoption of IHR (2005), see Chapter 2). Thus, the language surrounding discourses of global health highlights specific dimensions of risk, which emphasize concerns with global economic growth along with the security of world populations (Fidler 2011; Price-Smith 2009). Knowledge of the politico-economic context within which the avian influenza outbreak occurred in Thailand is necessary to understand how the risk of avian influenza turning pandemic was framed, which subsequently influenced the perception and management of risk.

The Experience of Risk Managers and the Availability of Control Options: The 2009 Swine Influenza Pandemic

In the midst of debates on the risk of a human pandemic, the 2009 H1N1 influenza pandemic was a timely litmus test for scientific and political judgement. As Chapter 10 will discuss, the global spread of H1N1 provided an opportunity to validate different approaches to risk assessment, while subjecting local policies of disease control to international scrutiny. Two months after the virus was first isolated, WHO declared a pandemic phase six (WHO 2009), the highest alert level on the pandemic risk assessment scale. However, when the pandemic turned out to be relatively moderate (Nicoll and McKee 2010), many observers argued that WHO had overstated its warning and control recommendations and generated unnecessary confusion and fear at the global level (Doshi 2011). WHO's controversial decision to change the definition of pandemic just after the novel strain of H1N1 was identified, and the refusal to disclose the names of the experts who were responsible for risk assessment, added to the controversy (Cohen and Carter 2010; Collignon 2009; Lynn 2010; Spiegel 2010).

In these debates, attention has been paid to the ways in which WHO risk assessment might have been affected by the experience of its managers. The 1918 Spanish influenza, for instance, was often quoted in policy speeches, scientific journals and the media on the prospect of another H1N1 pandemic influenza by way of analogy and extrapolation (Eggo et al. 2011; Honigsbaum 2009; Morens and Fauci 2007; Taubenberger and Morens 2006; Vynnycky et al. 2007), despite inconsistent documentation on the former. Likewise, the Asian influenza of 1957 and the Hong Kong influenza of 1968 remain prominent historical references to inform policy strategy. To deal with the inherent uncertainties of pandemic risk, past experiences and information about what an influenza pandemic is, and its likely consequences, are routinely used as a reference model for producing risk assessments. This process may be further enhanced when risk managers have personal first-hand experience with past episodes of severe epidemics (Heimer 1988). It is no coincidence, perhaps, that some of the key influenza experts who raised the alert level during the 2009 pandemic episode had formerly been involved in managing the aggressive strain of avian influenza H5N1 in Hong Kong, including the WHO Director-General Dr Margaret Chan.

Clearly, historical evidence and personal experiences can be inappropriate in non-routine situations when blindly extrapolated, especially in predicting the occurrence of a rare event (Fineberg 2009; Walch and Ungson 1991). In the case of the 2009 influenza pandemic, the assumption and anticipation of a clinically severe pandemic, subsequently challenged by its relatively moderate impact, begets a re-examination of the risk perceptions of managers involved in pandemic influenza policy and planning.

In addition, it is possible that the availability of an effective influenza vaccine may have further distorted risk perception (Fineberg 2009, Kahn 2009). When the first outbreaks of avian influenza H5N1 occurred, control options to prevent and mitigate the impact of a potential H5N1 pandemic were limited – a situation that led health authorities to prioritize containment over mitigation strategies (Lugner and Postma 2009). By contrast, well before the first pandemic stages in 2009, many high-income countries had 'sleeping' contracts with pharmaceutical companies to purchase H1N1 influenza vaccine should a pandemic occur. The availability of a vaccine prototype during the 2009 pandemic could have strengthened the risk perception that an influenza pandemic was imminent (Hine 2010). Thus, the availability of control options can lead to different policy strategies and outcomes. In the case of high- income countries, access to an influenza vaccine might have overvalued the perceptible cost of not attending to the risk, leading to justifications of a precautionary public health approach (Commission of the European Communities 2000). On the other hand, in resource-limited countries, the perception of risk may be present but framed differently (Durodie 2009; Wildavsky and Dake 1990), such as in terms of national economic interest and global inequalities.

A Conceptual Framework

The analysis of these three cases (swine influenza [1976], H5N1 [2004] and H1N1 [2009]) can inform the development of a conceptual framework on risk, which is graphically illustrated in Figure 3.1.

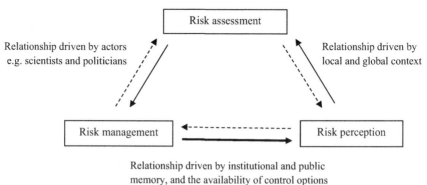

Figure 3.1   A conceptual framework on risk characterisation

Our proposed conceptual framework assumes a cyclical view (Gerrard and Petts 1998), with the solid lines representing the direction and relationship between the sub-concepts of risk assessment, risk perception and risk management. In this framework, risk perception influences risk assessment, which in turn influences risk management. This is well illustrated by the 1976 swine influenza scare, where the perception of a long overdue human influenza pandemic led to an unfavourable risk assessment and the subsequent hasty intervention of politicians in a bid to forestall the pandemic.

In addition, the dotted lines represent the interactive dynamic between the three components as evident in the actual practice of risk management in the three case studies that we have examined. The framing of the avian influenza risk in Thailand suggests that perceptions of pandemic risk can be influenced by questions of economic interest that are not necessarily related to the aim of protecting populations from public health threats. It is therefore not always the case that risk perception feeds into risk assessment, as the opposite pattern may also occur. Finally, the bold line represents the feedback loop evident during the 2009 influenza pandemic, where past risk management experiences shaped current risk perceptions, which then influenced how the pandemic risk was finally assessed and managed.

Discussion and Conclusion

This chapter examined the concept and practice of risk management in relation to pandemic influenza policy and control. As the analysis of the three case studies illustrates, risk assessment must be seen in a context of complex interdependencies with elements of risk perception and risk management. In all cases, the assessment of pandemic risk was subjected not only to the epistemic uncertainties of predictive knowledge, but also to political and economic imperatives, local and international contexts, the individual experiences of risk managers, and the availability of control options. This brings us back full circle to the concerns laid out in Chapter 1 – surveillance (which informs risk perception and risk assessment) occurs in a political context. Understanding the reasons why certain risks are at the forefront of the public agenda at a specific point in time reveals the deeper social structures, relationships and conditions that produce the 'visible surface' of public health interventions (Farmer 1996; McMichael 1995). The issue of how risk is assessed, perceived and managed, and whether there are substantive grounds for specific policy options, is particularly critical in the area of pandemic influenza policy and control, given the limitation of resources, especially in less developed countries.

Thus, our conceptual framework can help raise policy-makers' awareness of the inherent difficulties of risk assessment as it relates to risk management as well as the potential pitfalls of biased risk perception in decision-making. The over-reliance on conventional modelling tools in risk assessment alone can narrow the scope of risk analysis and range of risk management decisions (Farmer 1996). While a reductionist approach towards risk assessment may help the scientist and politician in dealing with real-life complexity by focusing on aspects assumed to be critical in decision-making, such an approach may overlook important input parameters (Focardi and Jonas 1998; Stiglitz et al. 2009). This may result in interventions that poorly address the risk at hand. Decision-making then becomes susceptible to an assessment tool based on mistaken premises and can potentially be jeopardized by considerations other than public health.

In addition, the scientific community may be more cognizant of its methods and role as the provider of risk analyses to policy-makers and the public (Freudenburg 1996). Although social scientists have challenged the exclusive priority given to quantitative methods and produced alternative understandings of risk based on interests, power relations and cultural perceptions (Douglas and Wildavsky 1983), quantitative methods are likely to remain predominant in the field of risk assessment; to venture into the other continuum with qualitative methods is likely to be more problematic, due to potential problems of reliability and validity. The advocate proposition of 'bridging two cultures of risk analysis' is persuasive and topical (Jasanoff 1993), but combining both approaches in public health policy is difficult. Over the past few years, the so-called 'One World, One Health' movement has called for more holistic approaches to policy research on communicable diseases, including the contribution of various disciplines and perspectives. However, the integration of different methodologies, metric systems and theoretical frameworks into a coherent system for risk assessment and management presents important challenges, both in professional and methodological terms. For example, recent contributions demonstrated that the study of health risks in epidemiology, despite claims to disciplinary 'openness', is rather based on an impermeable set of theoretical and methodological assumptions (Amsterdamska 2005; Farmer 1996; McMichael 1995). Yet, interdisciplinarity is much needed in risk assessment and management to fill the knowledge gaps between quantitative and qualitative methodologies. Predicting future trends of highly uncertain phenomena such as epidemics is a daunting, almost impossible task; however, understanding the social and cultural complexities of the societies in which associated risks are perceived and framed brings us closes to addressing these implementation gaps.

Acknowledgements

The authors are grateful for the London School of Hygiene and Tropical Medicine (LSHTM) School Trust Funds sponsorship.

References

Adams, J. 1995. *Risk*. London: University College of London.

Amsterdamska, O. 2005. Demarcating Epidemiology. *Science, Technology, Human Values*, 30 (1), 17–51.

Atun, R. and Gurol-Urganci, I. 2005. Health Expenditure: An 'Investment' Rather Than a Cost? *The Royal Institute of International Affairs*. Available at: http://www.chathamhouse.org/publications/papers/view/108071 [Accessed: 4 July 2011].

Aveyard, H. 2007. *Doing a Literature Review in Health and Social Care*. New York, NY: Open University Press.

BBC. 2005. Bird Flu Could Kill 150m People. *BBC News* [Online, 30 September] Available at: http://news.bbc.co.uk/2/hi/asia-pacific/4292426.stm [Accessed: 10 July 2011].

Beck, S. 2009. When Politics, and Swine Flu, Infect Health. *San Francisco Chronicle* [Online, 30 April] Available at: http://www.sfgate.com/opinion/article/When-politics-and-swine-flu-infect-health-3243724.php [Accessed: 9 August 2011].

Bloomberg. 2004. Fears of New Crisis: Sharp Rise in Bird Flu Cases in Thailand. *Bloomberg News Service* [Online, 18 April] Available at: http://poultry. information.in.th/bird-flu-archive-2004-july.html [Accessed: 5 July 2011].

Centers for Disease Control and Prevention. 2011. Researchers Reconstruct 1918 Pandemic Influenza Virus; Effort Designed to Advance Preparedness. *CDC Media Division* [Online, 5 October] Available at: http://www.cdc.gov/media/ pressrel/r051005.htm [Accessed: 10 July 2011].

Chan, M. 2006. Pandemic Flu: Communicating the Risks. *Bulletin of the World Health Organization*, 84 (1), 1–80.

Chompook, P., Sa, J.D., Hanvoravongchai, P., et al. 2009. *Thailand: Health System and Pandemic Preparedness*. Communicable Diseases Policy Research Group, London School of Hygiene and Tropical Medicine.

Cohen, D. and Carter, P. 2010. WHO and the Pandemic Flu 'Conspiracies'. *British Medical Journal*, 340, 2912–26.

Collignon, P. 2009. Take a Deep Breath, Swine Flu is Not that Bad. *Australas Emergency Nursing Journal*, 12, 71–2.

Commission of the European Communities 2000. *Communication from the Commission on the Precautionary Principle* [Online, 2 February] Available at: http://ec.europa.eu/dgs/health_consumer/library/pub/pub07_en.pdf [Accessed: 6 August 2011].

Cooper, H.M. 1982. Scientific Guidelines for Conducting Integrative Research Reviews. *Review of Educational Research*, 52 (2), 291–302.

Crouchy, M., Galai D. and Mark, R. 2006. Risk Management Á: A Helicopter View, in *The Essentials of Risk Management*, edited by M. Crouhy, D. Galai and R. Mark. New York: McGraw-Hill, 1–36.

Cunha, B.A. 2004. Influenza: Historical Aspects of Epidemics and Pandemics. *Infectious Disease Clinics of North America*, 18 (1), 141–55.

Doshi, P. 2011. The Elusive Definition of Pandemic Influenza. *WHO Bulletin*, 89, 532–8.

Douglas, M. and Wildavsky, A. 1983. *Risk and Culture*. Berkeley, CA: University of California Press.

Dowdle, W. 1997. The 1976 Experience. *The Journal of Infectious Diseases*, 176 (1), 69–72.

Durodie, B. 2004. The Limitations of Risk Management: Dealing with Disasters. *Tidsskriftet Politik*, 8 (1), 1–21.

Durodie, B., 2009. *Risk Perception and Communication*, NTS-Asia National Convention, Singapore, 3–4 November 2009, Available at: http://www. rsis-ntsasia.org/activities/conventions/2009-singapore/Bill%20Durodie.pdf [Accessed: 4 July 2011].

Eggo, R.M., Cauchemez, S. and Ferguson, N.M. 2011. Spatial dynamics of the 1918 Influenza Pandemic in England, Wales and the United States. *Journal of the Royal Society Interface*, 8 (55), 233–43.

Farmer, P. 1996. Social Inequalities and Emerging Infectious Diseases. *Emerging Infectious Diseases*, 2 (4), 259–69.

Ferguson, N. 2007. Capturing Human Behaviour. *Nature*, 446, 733.

Fidler, D.P. 2005. From International Sanitary Conventions to Global Health Security: The New International Health Regulations. *Chinese Journal of International Law*, 4 (2), 325–92.

_____. 2011. Assessing the Foreign Policy and Global Health Initiative: The Meaning of the Oslo Process. *The Royal Institute of International Affairs*. Available at: http://www.ghd-net.org/health-and-foreign-policy/assessing-foreign-policy-and-global-health-initiative-meaning-oslo-process [Accessed: 4 July 2011].

Fineberg, H. 2009. Swine Flu of 1976: Lessons from the Past. *Bulletin of the World Health Organization*, 87, 414–15.

Fineberg, H. and Neustadt, R., 1978. The swine flu affair: Decision-making on a slippery slope. Washington, DC: US Government Printing Office.

Focardi, S. and Jonas, C. 1998. Why Manage Risk? In *Risk Management: Framework, Methods, and Practice*, edited by S. Focardi and C. Jonas. New Hope, PA: John Wiley and Sons, 1–20.

Freudenburg, W.R. 1996. Risky Thinking: Irrational Fears about Risk and Society. *Annals of the American Academy of Political and Social Science*, 545, 44–53.

Gerrard, S. and Petts, J. 1998. Isolation or Integration? The Relationship Between Risk Assessment and Risk Management, in *Risk Assessment and Risk Management*, edited by R.E. Hester and R.M. Harrison. Cambridge: The Royal Society of Chemistry, 1–7.

Green, J. and Thorogood, N. 2004. *Qualitative Methods for Health Research*. London: Sage Publications.

Golafshani, N. 2003. Understanding Reliability and Validity in Qualitative Research. *The Qualitative Report*, 8 (4), 597–607.

Heimer, C.A. 1988. Social Structure, Psychology, and the Estimation of Risk. *Annual Review of Sociology*, 14, 491–519.

Hine, D.D. 2010. *The 2009 Influenza Pandemic: An Independent Review of the UK Response to the 2009 Influenza Pandemic*. Office of the Prime Minister and Cabinet: Pandemic Flu Response Review Team [Online, 1 July] Available at: http://www.cabinetoffice.gov.uk/resource-library/independent-review-response-2009-swine-flu-pandemic [Accessed: 10 July 2011].

Honigsbaum, M. 2009. Swine Flu: How Afraid Should We Be? The Telegraph [Online, 2 May] Available at: http://www.telegraph.co.uk/health/swine-flu/5264014/Swine-flu-How-afraid-should-we-be.html [Accessed: 5 July 2011].

Howard-Jones, N. 1975. The Scientific Background of the International Sanitary Conferences, 1851–1938. *Journal of the American Medical Association*, 235 (5), 514.

Jasanoff, S. 1993. Bridging the Two Cultures of Risk Analysis. *Risk Analysis*, 3 (2), 123–9.

Kahn, R. 2009. Will Avian Influenza Lead to a Human Pandemic? *The Journal of the European Medical Writers Association*, 18 (1), 29–31.

Lincoln, Y.S. and Guba, E.G. 1985. *Naturalistic Inquiry*. Beverly Hills, CA: Sage Publications.

Lugner, A.K. and Postma, M.J. 2009. Investment Decisions in Influenza Pandemic Contigency Planning: Cost-effectiveness of Stockpiling in Antiviral Drugs. *European Journal of Public Health*, 19 (5), 516–20.

Lynn, J. 2010. WHO to Review its Handling of H1N1 Flu Pandemic. *Reuters* [Online, 12 January] Available at: http://www.reuters.com/article/2010/01/12/us-flu-who-idUSTRE5BL2ZT20100112 [Accessed: 6 August 2011].

Mansnerus, E. 2010. Silence of Evidence in the Case of Pandemic Influenza Risk Assessment. *Centre for Analysis of Risk and Regulation, London School of Economics and Political Science*. Available at: http://eprints.lse.ac.uk/33101/ [Accessed: 3 July 2011].

Market Research Media. 2011. *Global Pandemic Influenza Preparedness Market Forecast 2010–2015* [Online] Available at: http://www.marketresearchmedia.com/?p=21 [Accessed: 6 August 2011].

McMichael, A.J. 1995. The Health of Persons, Populations, and Planet: Epidemiology Comes Full Circle. *Epidemiology and Society*, 6 (6), 633–6.

Menon, K.U. 2008. Risk Communications: In Search of a Pandemic. *Annals of Academy Medicine Singapore*, 37 (6), 525–34.

Menon, K.U. 2011. Pigs, People and a Pandemic: Communication Risk in a City-state. *Centre for Non-Traditional Security Studies, Nanyang Technological University*. Available at: http://www.rsis.edu.sg/NTS/resources/research_papers/NTS_Working_Paper6.pdf [Accessed: 3 July 2011].

Mintz, A. and Redd, S. 2003. Framing Effects in International Relations. *Synthese*, 135 (2), 193–213.

Moore, P.G. 1977. The Manager's Struggle with Uncertainty. *Journal of the Royal Statistical Society*, 140 (2), 129–65.

Morens, D.M. and Fauci, A.S. 2007. The 1918 Influenza Pandemic: Insights for the 21st Century. *Journal of Infectious Diseases*, 195 (7), 1018–28.

Nicita, A. 2007. Avian Influenza and the Poultry Trade. *World Bank* [Online, March] Available at: https://openknowledge.worldbank.org/handle/10986/6557 [Accessed: 28 June 2011].

Nicoll, A. and Mckee, M. 2010. Moderate Pandemic, Not Many Dead: Learning the Right Lessons in Europe from the 2009 Pandemic. *European Journal of Public Health*, 20 (5), 486–9.

Olsen, K. and Harvey, M. 2005. Asia-Pacific APEC Leaders Ready to Tackle Regional Issues: Focus Shifts to Flu Fear. *Dow Jones Reuters Business Interactive* [Online, 18 November].

Palese, P. 2004. Influenza: Old and New Threats. *Nature Medicine Supplement*, 10 (12), 82–7.

Patton, M.Q. 2002. *Qualitative Research and Evaluation Methods*. Thousand Oaks, CA: Sage Publications.

Perrin, A., 2004. Playing Chicken with Bird Flu [Online]. *Time Magazine*. Available at: http://www.time.com/time/magazine/article/0,9171,582473,00.html [Accessed: 28 June 2011].

Porter, T.M. 1995. *Trust in Numbers: The Pursuit of Objectivity in Science and Public Life*. New Jersey: Princeton University Press.

Price-Smith, A. 2009. *Contagion and Chaos: Disease, Ecology, and National Security in the Era of Globalization*. London: MIT Press.

Renn, O. and Rohrmann, B. 2000. The Concept of Risk, in *Cross-cultural Risk Perception: A Survey of Empirical Studies*, edited by O. Renn and B. Rohrmann. Dordrecht: Springer, 13–15.

Rip, A. 1986. The Mutual Dependence of Risk Research and Political Context. *Science & Technology Studies*, 4 (3/4), 3–15.

Safman, R. 2009. The Political Economy of Avian Influenza in Thailand. *STEPS Centre*. Available at: http://steps-centre.org/publication/the-political-economy-of-avian-influenza-in-thailand/ [Accessed: 3 July 2011].

Scoones, I. and Forster, P. 2010. Unpacking the International Response to Avian Influenza: Actors, Networks and Narratives, in *Avian Influenza: Science, Policy and Politics*, edited by I. Scoones. London: Earthscan, 19–64.

Siegel, M. 2006. Bird flu II: Panic is the Real Danger. *International Herald Tribune* [Online, 18 March], 6

Spiegel. 2010. Reconstruction of a Mass Hysteria: The Swine Flu Panic of 2009. *Spiegel Online International* [Online, 3 December] Available at: http://www.spiegel.de/international/world/0,1518,682613,00.html [Accessed: 4 July 2011].

Stiglitz, J., Sen, A. and Fitoussi, J.P. 2009. *Report by the Commission on the Measurement of Economic Performance and Social Progress*. Paris: Commission on the Measurement of Economic Performance and Social Progress.

Tangwisutijit, N. 2005. Awaiting the Scourge. *The Nation*, 19 April, 1–3.

Taubenberger, J.K. and Morens, D.M. 2006. The 1918 influenza: The Mother of All Pandemics. *Emerging Infectious Diseases*, 12 (1), 15–22.

Tesh, S.N. 1988. *Hidden Arguments: Political Ideology and Disease Prevention Policy*. New Jersey: Rutgers University Press.

The Nation. 2004a. Thaksin's Message: 'United and Eat Chicken'. *The Nation*, 8 February, 1–2.

The Nation. 2004b. The Second Wave: Authorities Continue to Offer Premature Reassurances that Bird-flu Virus has been Contained. *The Nation*, 11 November, 1–2.

Tiensin, T., Chaitaweesub, P., Songserm, T., et al. 2005. Highly Pathogenic Avian Influenza H5N1, Thailand. *Emerging Infectious Diseases*, 11, 1661–72.

Tierney, K.J. 1999. Towards a Critical Sociology of Risk. *Sociology Forum*, 14 (2), 215–42.

Timpka, T., Eriksson, H., Gursky, E.A., et al. 2009. Population-based Simulations of Influenza Pandemics: Validity and Significance for Public Health Policy. *Bulletin of the World Health Organization*, 87 (4), 305–11.

UK Health Protection Agency. 2011. *Risk Assessment* [Online] Available from: http://www.hpa.org.uk/ProductsServices/ChemicalsPoisons/ChemicalRiskAssessment/RiskAssessment [Accessed: 10 July 2011].

US Environmental Protection Agency. 2011. *About Human Health Research at the Environmental Protection Agency* [Online] Available from: http://www. epa. gov/hhrp/about.html [Accessed: 8 August 2011].

Vynnycky, E., Trindall, A. and Mangtani, P. 2007. Estimates of the Reproduction Numbers of Spanish Influenza Using Morbidity Data. *International Journal of Epidemiology*, 36 (4), 881–9.

Walch, J.P. and Ungson, G.R. 1991. Organisational Memory. *The Academy of Management Review*, 16 (1), 57–91.

Walt, G. and Gilson, L. 1994. Reforming the Health Sector in Developing Countries: The Central Role of Policy Analysis. *Health Policy and Planning*, 9, 353–70.

Wildavsky, A. and Dake, K. 1990. Theories of Risk Perception: Who Fears What and Why? *Journal of the American Academy of Arts and Sciences*, 119 (4), 41–60.

World Bank. 2008. Evaluating the Economic Consequences of Avian Influenza [Online]. Available at: http://siteresources.worldbank.org/EXTAVIANFLU/ Resources/EvaluatingAHIeco nomics_2008.pdf [Accessed: 6 August 2011].

WHO. 2006. Epidemiology of WHO-confirmed Human Cases of Avian Influenza A(H5N1) Infection. *Weekly Epidemiological Record* [Online, 30 June] Available at: http://www.who.int/csr/don/2006_06_30/en/index.html [Accessed: 14 August 2011].

WHO. 2008. Cumulative Number of Confirmed Human Cases of Avian Influenza A/(H5N1) Reported to WHO. 16 December 2008. Available at: http://www. who.int/csr/disease/avian_influenza/country/cases_table_2008_12_16/en/ [Accessed: 18 December 2011].

WHO. 2009. World Now at the Start of 2009 Influenza Pandemic. *Statement to the press by WHO Director-General Dr Margaret Chan* [Online, 11 June] Available at: http://who.int/mediacentre/news/statements/2009/h1n1_pandemic_ phase6_20090611/en/index.html [Accessed: 3 August 2011].

Chapter 4

Biosurveillance, Human Rights, and the Zombie Plague

Jeremy R. Youde

When an infectious disease outbreak occurs, the international community has a moral and international legal obligation to track its spread and use the data collected for the benefit of the general population. Under the terms of the International Health Regulations (2005), the World Health Organization (WHO) is legally empowered to collect and disseminate biosurveillance data, and WHO's 194 Member-States are legally obligated to provide this data as one of their core public health functions and use it in a way that respects and promotes human rights. Human rights and biosurveillance have a complicated relationship with one another. On the one hand, surveillance systems are necessary in order to arrest the spread of infectious disease outbreaks so as to better protect the health of all communities. On the other hand, though, these same surveillance systems can be used in discriminatory ways, impose heavy burdens, and abrogate freedom of movement and speech. Is some sort of resolution or detente possible?

In this chapter, I investigate how the International Health Regulations (2005) empower WHO to operationalize biosurveillance in a manner that promotes and respects human rights as a transnational good that can benefit humanity as a whole. While this represents a significant step forward for the international community and better integrates biosurveillance and human rights, there remain some ambiguities and underdeveloped protections that deserve greater attention from the World Health Organization.

The real test of any relationship between biosurveillance and human rights, though, comes when it is pushed to its limits. Perhaps no transnational infectious disease outbreak could challenge the international community more than a zombie outbreak. The recent explosion of interest in zombies in popular culture (and academia) "provides a window into the subliminal or unstated fears of citizens, and zombies are no different" (Drezner 2010: 4). How well would the relationship between biosurveillance and human rights hold in the face of an outbreak of the undead?

To make this argument, I begin by examining the meaning of biosurveillance. This leads into a discussion of zombies and how representations of zombies in popular culture mirror infectious disease outbreaks. I then move on to explore how this idea has played out in the International Health Regulations (IHR). This treaty, the leading health-related treaty in the international community, has witnessed dramatic evolutions in its conceptualization of biosurveillance and the role of human rights. Finally, I examine how the interplay between respecting human rights and drawing on the resources and skills of non-state actors can encourage compliance with the International Health Regulations and safeguarding individual rights. The International Health Regulations' approach to human rights is not perfect, but its current form is a significant improvement over the past.

Defining Biosurveillance

What does it mean to talk about surveillance within the realm of global public health? With the passage of World Health Assembly Resolution WHA 58.3 in 2005, WHO clearly defined surveillance as:

> the systematic ongoing collection, collation, and analysis of data for public health purposes and the timely dissemination of public health information for assessment and public health response as necessary. (WHO 2005)

Three elements of this definition are key. First, this definition of surveillance emphasizes the role of aggregate data and a macro-level focus on statistical anomalies over particular individuals or individual cases. Individuals are important only insofar as they manifest a particular disease; it is the emergence and distribution of the disease itself that matters.

Second, because of its aggregate focus and need for extensive amounts of data to detect statistical anomalies, surveillance efforts are ongoing and encompass essentially the entire population at hand. If the emergence of any new disease or a change in its distribution occurs at random, then operations need to be in place at all times in order to allow the surveillance mechanisms to detect these changes.

Third, information in and of itself is less important than being able to act on it. This surveillance is intended for a specific purpose, and, as such, there need to be structures in place to act on the anomalies detected. This suggests the need for a robust public health infrastructure at subnational, national, and international levels to share information with relevant parties and take the appropriate actions to respond in a timely fashion.

WHA58.3's definition of surveillance provides the clearest understanding of how the World Health Organization conceptualizes biosurveillance and its relationship to it in the case of infectious diseases. Furthermore, it feeds into the surveillance requirements that exist in the International Health Regulations (2005).

Zombies and Infectious Disease

Simply put, zombies are the reanimated undead. They feast on the flesh and brains of living humans. While earlier origin myths posit that zombies are under the control of sorcerers (Davis 1988) or rise from the dead to avenge a crime committed against them during their lives (Davis 1997), modern zombies are "mindless monsters who do not feel pain and who have an immense appetite for human flesh. Their aim is to kill, eat, or infect people" (Munz et al. 2009: 136).

The similarities between zombies and infectious disease are quite extensive. Drezner calls zombies "an obvious metaphor for medical maladies" (2010: 4–5), and institutions like the University of Florida and the US Centers for Disease Control and Prevention (CDC) have created zombie apocalypse response plans as part of their pandemic preparation strategies (CDC 2011; Ybarra 2009). Three criteria demonstrate why zombieism makes an effective tool for understanding infectious disease outbreaks and pandemic preparations. First, the zombie plague passes person-to-person and via intimate contact. While there may exist animal reservoirs, the zombie virus exhibits sustained transmission among humans. Zombieism is not an airborne pathogen. Rather, it spreads when a zombie bites an uninfected person (Munz 2009: 136). Most depictions suggest that the virus is highly (if not inevitably) contagious and that zombies are inherently driven to infect others (for example, see *28 Days Later* [2002]; Brooks 2006; *Dawn of the Dead* [2004]; *Shaun of the Dead* [2004]; Webb and Byrnand 2008: 84).

Second, as with the outbreak of any novel pathogen, the origins of zombieism are generally unknown at the epidemic's beginning. The novelty of the disease, along with its mysterious origins, complicates attempts to stop its spread or find a cure. Potential origins of zombieism include mutations from animal viruses (*28 Days Later* [2002]; *Dead Rising* [2006]) and fallout from nuclear radiation (*Night of the Living Dead* [1968]), but many films and books openly acknowledge that they have only a limited understanding of the origins of the zombie epidemic (*Dawn of the Dead* [2004]; *Shaun of the Dead* [2004]). This parallels the SARS epidemic—a disease whose origins remain clouded in mystery today.[1]

Finally, most depictions of zombie outbreaks portray an existential threat to the continued existence of society and civilization as we know it.[2] The film *Zombieland* (2009) opens with the main character lamenting the United States' destruction because of rampant zombieism. *World War Z* describes a post-apocalyptic world in which previous forms of political and economic organization are largely non-existent (Brooks 2006). From a more academic perspective, Munz and his co-authors employ statistical modeling techniques to argue that a zombie outbreak would be disastrous and "likely lead to the collapse of civilization" (2009: 146). While this may appear overblown, it mirrors the predictions of the effects of an influenza epidemic on the scale of 1918 in today's world. With a widespread outbreak, Osterholm (2005) envisions a world in which border security is prioritized to prevent non-citizens from accessing treatment and roving

---

1   Theories for SARS' emergence have linked the disease to bats, civets, and even extraterrestrial bacteria. See Lovgren (2003).

2   One notable exception is *Shaun of the Dead*, in which zombies come to play an important role in society by performing manual labor and competing on game shows.

bands of militias fill the void left by the breakdown in law and order. In 2006, Anne-Marie Slaughter likened an avian flu outbreak to a nuclear strike on a city because both "could kill millions" and "completely disrupt the way we live our lives" (cited in Quiñones 2006). Thus, the consequences of a zombie outbreak in many ways reflect the discussions among some policy advisors when responding to disease outbreaks.

Surveillance under IHR (2005)

As noted in chapters 1 and 2, the microbial world of 1969, when the previous version of the International Health Regulations was written, was fundamentally different from that of 2005.

IHR (2005) fundamentally transformed biosurveillance in four key ways. First, the new Regulations embrace an "all risks" approach (Fidler and Gostin 2006). This approach significantly broadened the scope of biosurveillance operations. Instead of identifying specific diseases, IHR (2005) require states to report "all events which may constitute a public health emergency of international concern within its territory" (Article 6). They further define a "public health emergency of international concern" (PHEIC) as "extraordinary event which ... constitute[s] a public health risk to other States through the international spread of disease and ... potentially require[s] a coordinated international response" (Article 1). National governments must assess an outbreak's severity within 48 hours of initial detection and send a report to WHO within 24 hours of confirmation (Sturtevant 2007: 118). This report should include case definitions, laboratory findings, morbidity and mortality incidents, risk factors, and initial public health responses.

Second, along with the reporting requirements, IHR (2005) mandate surveillance and reporting structures for states to stay in contact with WHO. Each state must designate a National IHR Focal Point that will be accessible at all times for communicating with the WHO (Article 1). The National IHR Focal Point must take responsibility for communicating with the appropriate offices at the WHO. Third, as noted in Chapter 1, IHR (2005) broadened the number and nature of parties that can report about public health emergencies to WHO. Under previous versions of the IHR, states were the only entities that could make reports to WHO. Non-state sources had no standing to report disease outbreaks—but now they do. These changes introduce a host of new eyes and ears to keep watch and hold governments accountable for their response to public health emergencies.

Fourth, IHR (2005) most notably—for the first time—explicitly recognize the need to consider and respect human rights in the context of dealing with public health emergencies. They recognize that the risks from infectious diseases are not only physical in nature, but can also negatively affect a person's political and social spheres. Earlier versions of the IHR made no mention of human rights. This potentially posed problems, as surveillance techniques and responses to public health emergencies often ignored existing human rights standards. Gostin

(2004: 2626) notes, "Infectious disease powers curtail individual freedoms, bodily integrity, and liberty. At the same time, public health activities can stigmatize, stereotype, or discriminate against individuals or groups." Governments would implement trade and travel restrictions in an arbitrary manner. Some would impose quarantine or isolation policies (Plotkin and Kimball 1997). Though IHR (2005) specified that its policies were the maximum allowed under international law, states often chose to violate this provision, knowing that WHO lacked the legal mechanisms to punish them for such transgressions (Calain 2007: 4). IHR (2005) still abide by the Siracusa Principles and their claim that states may temporarily limit rights to implement disease control measures (United Nations 1985), but they gave human rights a great boost within global health.

Human Rights in IHR (2005)

Between the IHR's original incarnation and its revisions that began in the 1990s, public health officials came to recognize the importance of human rights in implementing effective disease control strategies. Jonathan Mann pioneered much of this recognition, showing that HIV/AIDS strategies that respected and emphasized human rights were more successful than those that stigmatized HIV-positive persons (Mann et al. 1999). This growing acceptance of the importance of human rights within public health strategies convinced those rewriting the IHR to explicitly include human rights provisions in the revised Regulations. Six articles within IHR (2005) address human rights concerns:

- Article 3: implement IHR (2005) "with full respect for the dignity, human rights, and fundamental freedom of persons";
- Article 23: avoid subjecting travelers to medical examinations without their consent, and make any such examinations as minimally invasive as possible;
- Article 31: respect travelers' dignity, human rights, and fundamental freedoms;
- Article 42: implement IHR (2005) in a transparent, non-discriminatory manner;
- Article 43: allow states the right to implement their own disease control measures outside the formal IHR (2005) process, provided that they are generally consistent with the Regulations and no more intrusive than necessary;
- Article 45: keep personal data is anonymous and confidential, and retain such data only as long as necessary for its specific purpose.

By explicitly referencing human rights in a health-related context, IHR (2005) present a significant step forward toward realizing human rights on a broad scale. Unfortunately, the force of the human rights protections remains relatively underdeveloped. The rhetorical commitment does not come with an international legal commitment that is as vigorous. Whose human rights should be respected and the nature of those rights are surprisingly ambiguous, especially given the prominence of human rights treaties within the international law arena. The Regulations do call upon member-states to respect human rights, but they do so in a relatively passive manner. For instance, only Articles 3 and 31 explicitly use the term human rights. Even more curiously, the human rights-related articles stress the rights of travelers[3]—people passing through a country or staying temporarily—as opposed to explicitly protecting the human rights of a state's own citizens and residents. They do not provide the World Health Organization with the power to independently investigate claims of human rights abuses in the biosurveillance realm. The human rights articles are certainly an improvement over previous versions of the IHR—IHR (1969) contains no mention of human rights, freedom, or dignity—but their mention of human rights lacks much power behind it.

Curiously, IHR (2005)'s references to human rights fail to highlight any human rights treaties. This is especially puzzling in light of the trend during the 1990s and beyond toward greater acceptance of universal human rights and increasing internalization of those norms (Donnelly 2006: 11–16). The Constitution of the World Health Organization and the Charter of the United Nations, both referenced in Article 3, acknowledge the importance of human rights, but they provide little in terms of a framework or structure for their implementation—certainly far less than the myriad of subsequent human rights treaties that have emerged since then. The interaction between IHR (2005) and existing international human rights treaties remains largely unknown (Plotkin 2007: 844).

Being more explicit about human rights protections within IHR (2005) would encourage states to better integrate human rights thinking into their application of the Regulations. It would also encourage compliance with IHR (2005)'s mandates. People are more likely to report disease outbreaks if they know that they will not face punitive measures. If fears exist that expanded surveillance measures threaten to abrogate the rights of individuals or will be applied in a discriminatory manner, then it is vitally important that the increased surveillance comes with a vigorous and overt acknowledgement of the role of human rights.

Human Rights, Biosurveillance, and Zombies

To examine how well IHR (2005) would respond to a zombie outbreak, it helps to focus on the four innovations described above. First, IHR (2005)'s "all-risks" approach would include zombieism since the illness exhibits the characteristics that would necessitate reporting its outbreak to WHO. Using the four-question decision-making matrix provides the tools to determine whether zombieism constitutes a public health emergency of international concern. Popular depictions of zombieism demonstrate that it has a serious public health impact, qualifies as an

---

3   Plotkin (2007: 844) introduces a further complication, noting that "traveler" itself is an ambiguous term without a precise definition.

unusual or unexpected event, possesses a significant risk of international spread, and has the potential to cause serious interruptions to trade and travel. As such, IHR (2005) are in effect and WHO will have a central role to play in coordinating the response.

Second, IHR (2005) member-states must establish and maintain active surveillance and reporting structures to stay in contact with the World Health Organization. This means that states need the capabilities to find disease outbreaks within their own borders—not simply at the borders. Possessing a functioning surveillance system that looked at both internal and external sources of outbreaks would go a long way toward helping to stop an outbreak of zombieism before it got too out of control. The country's National IHR Focal Point would have a moral and international legal obligation to report the outbreak of zombieism to WHO, and it could not abdicate its responsibilities by arguing that it lacked active surveillance capacities. By being a party to IHR (2005), that state must acquire such capacities. WHO, regional WHO offices, and other organizations may help with the implementation, but it is ultimately the state's responsibility. Once a report is made, though, then WHO takes a leading role in collaboration with government officials.

Third, non-state actors have the right and ability to make reports to WHO, and WHO can act on those reports. Even if a state were unwilling or unable to implement and maintain a surveillance system sensitive enough to detect a novel disease outbreak like zombieism, IHR (2005) explicitly allows non-state actors to make reports of disease outbreaks to WHO. This has two important benefits for the international community. First, it would ensure that WHO receives the reports of zombieism in a timely manner—even if government officials resisted making such a report. This would allow WHO and others to mobilize faster. Second, it places an additional pressure on the state to make the report itself. Under the old system, a state that wanted to prevent information about a disease outbreak from getting to WHO for fear of the economic consequences, the hit to its reputation, or its national pride could effectively squelch the process. It is understandable why a government might want to prevent a report of zombieism from getting out. With IHR (2005), though, non-state actors could make reports even if the government did not want such information to get out. On the basis of that information, WHO could request the state to undertake an investigation. It could also mobilize its own forces to initiate a response. As Dr Guénäel Rodier, WHO's Director of IHR Coordination, stated, "In today's information society, you cannot ignore or hide a problem for very long. You can perhaps ignore or hide an event for a day or two, but after a week it's virtually impossible. WHO and its partners have a powerful system of gathering intelligence that will pick anything up immediately" (Rodier 2007: 428). In addition, reports about the zombieism outbreak could emerge through any number of internet-based surveillance systems, like ProMED Mail or BioCaster (for more information on these systems, see chapters 5 and 6). By expanding the reporting universe, IHR (2005) could induce states to be more forthcoming with reporting any cases of zombieism. States would have an incentive to make the report themselves instead of being shamed into responding. Allowing non-state actors could also prove helpful if the National IHR Focal Point were incapacitated (perhaps by having been bitten by a zombie or too fearful of the hordes of zombies surrounding the office) to report to WHO.

Finally, IHR (2005) explicitly mandates that states respect dignity and human rights when implementing disease control strategies. It is this last area where IHR (2005)'s lack of specificity may cause the most problems. Under IHR (2005), states are not to impose or introduce policies that violate the human rights and personal dignity of the affected. This does not explicitly rule out quarantine or isolation, but it does place an additional burden on states introducing such policies. Let us suppose that a governmental entity wanted to protect the uninfected by placing them in a single location where they could remain safe. If zombie movies have taught us anything, it is that people tend to flock to the indoor shopping mall for protection—and that this strategy almost inevitably fails. Under IHR (2005), simply corralling the uninfected into the mall would violate their rights and dignity unless they were also provided with the supplies necessary to ensure an adequate quality of life. Furthermore, the state would have a positive obligation to patrol the mall to ensure that no zombies could enter through an unlocked fire door, loading dock, or air vent. If a state were to introduce such a policy, it could do so only so long as that strategy was necessary, and it could not compel individuals outside the affected area to leave their homes unless scientific evidence proved its necessity.

While IHR (2005) offers these sorts of human rights protections, it fails to include any recourse for those who feel their human rights have been violated. No appeals process exists, so those sent to the mall to protect them from the zombie hordes lack formal mechanisms for challenging their detention. This could make people fear the surveillance systems that picked up on the zombieism outbreak in the first place, disinclining them toward cooperating with authorities and encouraging people to hide from the very systems that should ideally offer them protection. If people fear that they will be unnecessarily separated from their loved ones (including those who may be infected), they may be tempted to hide in the attic (a favorite hiding place in many zombie movies). On a macro level, WHO lacks mechanisms to investigate reports or claims of human rights violations. It cannot hold states accountable for upholding the human rights of their citizens when the organization does not have the investigatory capacity to examine state actions or receive reports of potential violations.

These shortcomings do not present insurmountable obstacles. At the state level, IHR (2005) could introduce an appeals process. Page suggests a legal procedure based on quarantine regulations in Canada and the rights of those involuntarily committed to psychiatric institutions in the American state of West Virginia. At its heart, Page's proposal would ensure access to the court system for those who find themselves subject to quarantine or wish to question elements of biosurveillance. Her approach mandates five guarantees to those subject to regulation due to biosurveillance or quarantine. First, the affected party would have the right to adequate written notice of the grounds for regulation or detention. Second, the affected party would have the right to counsel (or, if indigent, the right to have counsel provided for them). Third, the affected party would have the right to be present at any and all hearings and retain the right to cross-examine or question any witnesses that testified during the proceedings. Fourth, under this proposal, the standard for affirming the necessity of surveillance-related regulation or detention would be the existence of clear, cogent, and convincing evidence. Finally, the affected party would have the right to receive a written verbatim transcript of the proceedings for use in any appeals of the court's decision (Page 2006/2007: 524–5). Canadian law, which places the responsibility for establishing and enforcing quarantine regulations at the national level, uses a similar procedure. In addition, though, Canadian quarantine regulations explicitly provide for expedited judicial review for cases of involuntary detention. After being held for 48 hours, the Minister of Health must confirm a person's quarantine designation and forward that confirmation to a superior court judge in the affected person's province. The judge must then hear the case and make a decision about the appropriateness of the quarantine within one day. If the Minister of Health fails to inform a superior court judge of his or her order within two days of the initial 48 hours, the quarantined individual is free to leave. Page (2006/2007: 536) praises the Canadian approach for "appropriately balanc[ing] the rights of individuals" with broader societal concerns. This would present a way for those isolated in the mall to challenge the restrictions placed on them if they saw that as necessary.

On a broader level, the World Health Organization needs to find a way to engage in some measure of monitoring or investigation of reports of human rights violations. The IHR (2005) Review Committee advocated for WHO (2005: 82) to consult with state authorities when media reports suggested that human rights violations occurred. This arrangement would presumably be less formal than an actual investigation of human rights violations—something WHO lacks the resources or experiences to conduct on its own—but could still signal to states that their actions do receive notice. Indeed, it is on this latter point where unofficial sources can perhaps play their most useful role in encouraging compliance with and respect for human rights within biosurveillance procedures. Non-governmental organizations could monitor the policies introduced to keep the uninfected safe and treat the infected in accordance with recognized medical procedures for treating zombieism. Indeed, non-state actors could practically introduce a division of labor—a group like Human Rights Watch could make sure that the uninfected, who are still human, are not subject to arbitrary detention or discriminatory treatment, and a new organization like People for the Ethical Treatment of Zombies (PETZ) could ensure zombies are neither subject to medical experimentation without consent nor dispatched by a skilled sniper firing a single bullet into their brain.

These findings suggest that IHR (2005) can provide some useful tools for responding to a zombie plague. They encourage states to engage in active surveillance, allow for a wide variety of state and non-state sources to make reports of disease outbreaks, and explicitly recognize the importance and value of human rights in addressing a pandemic. That said, the human rights protections in particular remain relatively weak and undefined. The lack of specificity could unnecessarily introduce fear and wariness about the surveillance procedures and encourage people to evade disease control measures. Greater specificity could help overcome this problem and ensure that the international community stops the zombie outbreak before it has a chance to establish itself and threaten more people.

Taken altogether, these changes in the International Health Regulations (2005) elevate the stature of the World Health Organization in responding to infectious disease outbreaks like zombieism. While WHO cannot replace state functions, the treaty empowers it to take a far more active role. It also allows WHO to implement IHR (2005) as an international good, rather than narrowly focusing on trade, travel, and commercial concerns.

Conclusion

The revisions to the International Health Regulations in 2005 fundamentally remade the international community's most prominent health-related treaty. The treaty moved away from a syndrome-specific approach to biosurveillance to an expansive threat-based model. This necessarily required the expansion of surveillance activities, which can cause fear and consternation over the government's intentions. To allay some of those fears, though, IHR (2005), for the first time ever, explicitly integrated respect for human rights into its operating procedures. Furthermore, IHR (2005) provided avenues whereby non-state actors could contribute to disease reporting and to keeping an eye on a government's response to a disease outbreak. Combining respect for human rights and the inclusion of non-state actors has the potential to ensure the usefulness of IHR (2005) and to encourage compliance with the treaty's requirements. Non-state actors can play a vital role in assessing the sorts of activities in which governments engage in the name of disease control. With these changes, the IHR (2005) firmly entrenched WHO as the key recipient of biosurveillance data and empowered it to act on that information as appropriate. While the recognition of human rights within the treaty is significant, it would be useful to also empower the World Health Organization with the powers to oversee and ensure that human rights are being protected when these surveillance systems are put into practice.

With any luck, the human race will never experience an outbreak of zombieism. The consequences of such an epidemic could be far-reaching and traumatic. That said, history reminds us that the microbial world is ever-changing and unpredictable. Therefore, it behooves humanity to be ready to respond to such an outbreak. The International Health Regulations (2005) are the most far-reaching tools the international community possesses to respond to a zombie plague or any other infectious disease outbreak, and the treaty puts the World Health Organization at the center of that response.

References

28 Days Later [Movie]. 2002. Directed by Danny Boyle. DNA Films/British Film Council.

Baker, M.G. and Fidler, D.P. 2006. Global Public Health Surveillance under New International Health Regulations. *Emerging Infectious Diseases*, 12 (7), 1058–65.

Brooks, M. 2006. *World War Z: An Oral History of the Zombie War*. New York: Crown.

Calain, P. 2007. Exploring the International Arena of Global Public Health Surveillance. *Health Policy and Planning*, 22 (1), 2–12.

Centers for Disease Control and Prevention. 2011. *Preparedness 101: Zombie Apocalypse* [Online, Centers for Disease Control and Prevention] Available at: http://www.bt.cdc.gov/socialmedia/zombies_blog.asp [Accessed: 26 July 2011].

Davis, W. 1997. *The Serpent and the Rainbow: A Harvard Scientist's Astonishing Journey into the Secret Societies of Haitian Voodoo, Zombis, and Magic*. New York: Touchstone.

Davis, W. 1988. *Passage of Darkness: The Ethnobiology of the Haitian Zombie*. Chapel Hill, NC: University of North Carolina Press.

Dawn of the Dead [Movie]. 2004. Directed by Zach Snyder. Strike Entertainment.

Dead Rising [Video Game]. 2006. Produced by Keiji Inafune. Capcom.

Donnelly, J. 2006. *International Human Rights*. Boulder, CO: Westview Press.

Drezner, D.W. 2010. *Theories of International Politics and Zombies*. Princeton: Princeton University Press.

Fidler, D.P. and Gostin, L.O. 2006. The New International Health Regulations: An Historic Development for International Law and Public Health. *Journal of Medicine, Law, and Ethics*, 34 (1), 85–94.

Gostin, L.O. 2004. International Infectious Disease Law: Revision of the World Health Organization's International Health Regulations. *Health Law and Ethics*, 291 (21), 2623–7.

Lovgren, S. Far-out Theory Ties SARS Origins to Comet. *National Geographic News* [Online, 3 June] Available at: http://news.nationalgeographic.com/news/2003/06/0603_030603_sarsspace.html [Accessed: 26 July 2011].

Mack, E. 2006. The World Health Organization's New International Health Regulations: Incursion On State Sovereignty and Ill-Fated Response to Global Health Issues. *Chicago Journal of International Law*, 7 (1), 365–78.

Mann, J.M., Grodin, M.A., Gruskin, S. and Annas, G.J. 1999. *Health and Human Rights: A Reader*. New York: Routledge.

Munz, P., Hudea, I., Imad, J. and Smith, R.J. 2009. When Zombies Attack! Mathematical Modelling of an Outbreak of a Zombie Infection, in *Infectious Disease Modelling Research Progress*, edited by J.M. Tchuenche and C. Chikaya. Hauppauge, NY: Nova Science Publishers.

Night of the Living Dead [Movie]. 1968. Directed by George A. Romero. Image Ten.

Osterholm, M. 2005. Preparing for the Next Pandemic. *Foreign Affairs* 84 (4), 24–37.

Page, E.M. 2006/2007. Balancing Individual Rights and Public Safety During Quarantine: The US and Canada. *Case Western Reserve Journal of International Law*, 38 (3–4), 517–37.

Plotkin, B.J. and Kimball, A.M. 1997. Designing an International Policy and Legal framework for the Control of Emerging Infectious Diseases: First Steps. *Emerging Infectious Diseases*, 3 (1), 1–9.

Plotkin, B.J. 2007. Human Rights and other Provisions in the Revised International Health Regulations (2005). *Public Health*, 121 (11), 840–45.

Quiñones, E. 2006. Project Aims to "Kindle Debate" on U.S. National Security. *Princeton Weekly Bulletin* [Online, 16 October] Available at: http://www.princeton.edu/main/news/archive/S16/10/08A65/index.xml [Accessed: 26 July 2011].

Rodier, G.R. 2007. New Rules on International Public Health Security. *Bulletin of the World Health Organization*, 85 (6), 428–31.

Rodier, G., Greenspan, A.L., Hughes, J.M. and Heymann, D.L. 2007. Global Public Health Security. *Emerging Infectious Diseases*, 13 (10), 1447–52.

Shaun of the Dead [Movie]. 2004. Directed by Edgar Wright. StudioCanal.

Sturtevant, J.L., Anema, A. and Brownstein, J.S. 2007. The New International Health Regulations: Considerations for Global Public Health Surveillance. *Disaster Medicine and Public Health Preparedness*, 1 (2), 117–21.

United Nations. 1985. *Siracusa Principles on the Limitation and Derogation Provisions in the International Covenant on Civil and Political Rights*, UN Doc. E/CN.4/1985/4, Annex. Available at: http://www1.umn.edu/humanrts/instree/siracusaprinciples.html [Accessed: 22 May 2014).

Webb, J. and Byrnand, S. Some Kind of Virus: The Zombie as Body and as Trope. *Body and Society* 14 (2), 83–98.

Wilson, K., McDougall, C., Fidler, D.P. and Lazar, H. 2008. Strategies for Implementing the New International Health Regulations in Federal Countries. *Bulletin of the World Health Organization*, 86 (3), 215–20.

World Health Organization 2005. *International Health Regulations (2005)*. Geneva: WHO Press.

_____. 2005. *Revision of the International Health Regulations (2005)* [Online, Fifty-Eighth World Health Assembly, Geneva, Switzerland]. Available at: http://www.who.int/gb/ebwha/pdf_files/WHA58/A58_4-en.pdf [Accessed: 8 July 2011].

_____. 2011. *Implementation of the International Health Regulations (2005): Report of the Reporting Committee on the Functioning of the International Health Regulations (2005) in Relation to Pandemic H1N1 (2009)* [Online: Sixty-Fourth World Health Assembly, Geneva, Switzerland]. Available at: http://www.ghd-net.org/sites/default/files/A64_10-en.pdf [Accessed: 26 July 2011].

Ybarra, J. 2009. *Zombie Attack: Disaster Preparedness Simulation Exercise #5 (DR5)* [Online, University of Florida] Available at: http://www.astro.ufl.edu/~jybarra/zombieplan.pdf [Accessed: 26 July 2011].

Zombieland [Movie]. 2009. Directed by Ruben Fleischer. Relativity Media.

Chapter 5
GPHIN Phase 3:
One Mandate, Multiple Stakeholders

Abla Mawudeku, Philip AbdelMalik, Richard Lemay, and Louise Boily

Introduction

The pursuit of strong economies, trade, and civil societies has inadvertently had serious public health implications (Cash and Narasimhan 2000; Davies 2012). As the transformation to the First Industrial Revolution in the late 1700s transitioned through to the Third in the 1970s, countries increasingly realized the intertwined linkages between health and the economy (Gill and Law 1988). In turn, this realization facilitated significant advancements in public health.

During the First Industrial Revolution, a systematic approach to outbreak investigation was established (Tulchinsky and Varavikova 2009). The Second Industrial Revolution was seen as the period of scientific discovery and innovation that included the discovery of the germ theory of disease and the development of vaccines (Tulchinsky and Varavikova 2009). Innovation in computing and electronics was the focus of what some have referred to as the Third Industrial Revolution.[1] This period embraced new technological breakthroughs including the use of Internet technology and digitization of products (Cerny 1993). This has led to a new level of globalization in which free trade has liberalized global trading systems and resulted in increased interconnectedness and interdependence of peoples and countries (Beaglehole and Bonita 2009).

Implications for public health are apparent in this new era because of the increased flow of information along with goods and people. The high mobility of people across the world has increased the risk of disease spread as demonstrated during the SARS outbreak (Zacher and Keefe 2008). Similarly the complexity associated with the global food supply chain has increased the risks of unsafe foods (Food and Agriculture Organization and World Health Organization 2012). Fortunately, technological innovation has also enabled the news of disease outbreaks to be transmitted in minutes around the world. Examples of the

---

1 O'Brien and Williams (2013) refer to three industrial revolutions. The first (1760–1830) refers to the British Industrial Revolution and the emergence of mass manufacturing. The second (1870–1914) focuses on technology as the applied use of scientific knowledge. The third (1990–present) is focused on the transition to the information age

rapidity in which media disseminated information and in certain situations caused unnecessary panic were seen during the outbreak of cholera in Peru, plague in India and Ebola in Congo (Zacher and Keefe 2008).

The proliferation of information on the Internet and mass media has presented an opportunity to leverage such information and communication technologies to strengthen global health surveillance for re-emerging and emerging public health threats. It has paved the way for a new approach to and mechanism for conducting global health surveillance (Zacher and Keefe 2008). This has led to a new frontier in global public health surveillance that incorporates 'event-based surveillance': a non-traditional public health surveillance methodology that, to a large extent, relies on the monitoring of unstructured data gathered from various sources of intelligence (Paquet et al. 2006).

The Global Public Health Intelligence Network (GPHIN) is, as the name implies, a network for public health intelligence with an event-based surveillance system at its core. It contributed to the general modernization, utility, and transparency of global health surveillance by speeding and revitalizing international surveillance while weakening governments' secrecy and control of information about public health events of potential global concern (Burns 2006; Mykhalovskiy and Weir 2006).

This chapter gives an overview of how the GPHIN is integrated and operates within the Canadian national public health surveillance system, discusses GPHIN's value more broadly and offers insight on the road ahead.

The Global Public Health Intelligence Network

GPHIN is an early-warning and situational awareness network that aims to be an indispensable source for the early detection of potential public health threats worldwide and the ongoing real-time monitoring of events. It has an all-hazards approach, covering a broad spectrum of public health issues that include human, animal, zoonotic and plant diseases; biologics (e.g. vaccines); chemical, radiological and nuclear incidents; unsafe products and natural and man-made disasters.

Not every signal identified by GPHIN is necessarily the next SARS (Severe Acute Respiratory Syndrome); the intent of GPHIN is to provide an early warning to the World Health Organization (WHO) and other institutions of possible threats, necessitating further verification, communication, and follow-up action as appropriate. GPHIN is not designed or intended to be a pandemic foghorn, and the balance between the system's sensitivity and specificity is a delicate one that continues to be refined in the ever-changing economy of information sharing.

The network consists of three elements: an application to manage the data; a team of analysts and information technology (IT) specialists; and a network of users that can respond to the signals issued.

The GPHIN Application

Since GPHIN's genesis in 1998 as an event-based surveillance application, it has continued to evolve, taking advantage of the wealth of open-source data made available through advancements in information communication technologies (ICT).

The application is a secure, Internet-based and multilingual tool that continuously searches global media sources such as news wires and Web sites to identify information about disease outbreaks and other events of potential international public health concern. As a multilingual application, GPHIN monitors relevant public health events in nine languages: Arabic, Chinese (simplified and traditional), English, Farsi, French, Portuguese, Russian, and Spanish (Mawudeku et al. 2013). The automated computerized process assists the analysts by rapidly processing high volumes of daily news reports. An average of 20,000 reports are automatically processed daily, and approximately 2,000 to 4,000 of the reports that are considered relevant remain on the system for viewing. The processing includes a series of actions beginning with the identification and extraction of relevant news reports. Those that are considered to be duplicates are removed. The non-English news reports are then machine-translated to English and vice versa resulting in a 'gist' that delivers the essence of the content of the report. While the translation is not the same quality as that provided by professional translators, it does provide instantaneous translations at a lower cost. Using algorithms, the news reports are filtered for relevance, mined and classified based on the GPHIN's taxonomy and ontology, and prioritized by relevancy.

The relevant news and consequent situational awareness and public health intelligence reports generated by the analysts are accessible to the GPHIN membership, which has access to the GPHIN application through the Web on a 24/7 basis anywhere in the world where there is Internet access.

The GPHIN Analysts

The human analysis process is provided 18 hours per day, 6 days a week. However, during public health emergencies (e.g. SARS, Pandemic (H1N1) 2009, etc.), the analysts' responsibilities are extended to 24/7 coverage. This component entails a multidisciplinary team of analysts that draw on their linguistic, technical and analytical expertise to conduct rapid risk assessments and identify and flag emerging events that may have significant public health consequences. A Canada 'IHR-plus' decision tool is used to assess events and consists of established criteria based on the WHO International Health Regulations Annex 2 Decision Instrument (WHO 2008a; see Figure 1.1 in Chapter 1), coupled with additional criteria to help identify risks that are more specific to the Canadian context. The same tool using only the IHR criteria is used to assess if there are any potential risks to the international community.

To address the broad spectrum of public health issues captured by the GPHIN application, it is necessary for the team to have diverse knowledge across various disciplines that include public health, social sciences, natural and environmental sciences, medicine, surveillance, and journalism. The analysts also use various sources of information to assist with risk assessment. References include the WHO Global Health Observatory, WHO International Travel and Health, disease distribution maps, GLEWS Reports, FAO Databases and various historical data on diseases.

Responsibilities of the analysts also include but are not limited to the identification of trends or possible relationships between events. They are also responsible for the publication of situational awareness reports, improvements in the comprehensibility of machine translated news reports, and the construction and updating of search syntaxes and keywords used for the extraction and retrieval of relevant news reports.

The GPHIN Network

The GPHIN network membership spans public health institutions at the international and national levels. These include key stakeholders such as WHO, Food and Agriculture Organization (FAO), World Organisation for Animal Health (OIE), ministries of health, and other related public health departments.

The network has been a critical component of the GPHIN. During its pilot phase, the collaboration with WHO demonstrated the necessity for WHO to be an integral participant in the framework for gathering public health intelligence (Hitchcock et al. 2007; Davies 2008; Davies and Youde 2012). WHO has the mandate to monitor and verify global public health threats of international concern, which is a critical role (Grein et al. 2001). Similarly, FAO and OIE have combined efforts with the WHO under the establishment of the Global Early Warning System to detect, verify and respond to animal disease, including zoonoses (FAO, OIE, and WHO 2006). The absence of the participation of these international organizations in global surveillance would compromise the ability of State Parties to be able to verify any public health events of concern gleaned from unofficial reports (to read further on this point, see the H1N1 case in Chapter 2 and H5N1 case in Chapter 8).

Public Health Intelligence: The Canadian Model

The Public Health Agency of Canada (PHAC) is the federal agency that was established in 2004 following the evaluation of Canada's response to SARS and the recommendation to have an entity responsible for public health in Canada. A National Advisory Committee on SARS and Public Health (2003) was established by the Minister of Health in May 2003 to provide an independent assessment of current public health efforts and lessons learned from SARS (Public Health Agency of Canada Act 2006).

The agency, which was created out of the federal Department of Health, is responsible for the promotion and protection of the health of Canadians. Within the agency, various centres were established, among them the Centre for Emergency Preparedness and Response (CEPR) where GPHIN resides.

Over the years, several drivers have resulted in the expansion and restructuring of the Agency. In Canada, these have included the Emergency Management Act (Minister of Justice 2007) that outlines the federal role in emergency management and the integration of an All Hazards Risk Approach (Public Safety Canada 2011) for assessing the impact and likelihood of both malicious and non-malicious hazards and threats that Canada could face). Globally, the revised International Health Regulations (WHO 2008a) have also contributed to the Agency's transformation over the years.

In the Spring of 2013, the agency established the Health Security and Infrastructure Branch where CEPR is located. The Branch is essential for strengthening Canada's ability to establish the foundation pieces needed to build its health security capacity. HSIB was officially named on April 5 2013. The new branch serves as the Agency's central coordinating point on health security matters relating to public health capacity development, surveillance strategy and data management, emergency preparedness and response, and biosecurity. It is a shared service, thereby providing leadership and support to Canada's Health Portfolio (Health Canada, the Public Health Agency of Canada, the Canadian Food Inspection Agency, the Canadian Institutes of Health Research, the Hazardous Materials Information Review Commission, the Patented Medicine Prices Review Board, and Assisted Human Reproduction Canada) and other federal departments.

Today, GPHIN plays an integral role within CEPR and the Public Health Agency of Canada's daily operations. It is housed alongside Canada's International Health Regulations National Focal Point Office (IHR NFPO) within the Situational Awareness Section (SAS) under CEPR. SAS together with CEPR's Watch Office (the single window for operations centres at the federal, provincial and territorial levels to share information about emerging threats to Canadians that may have public health implications) form a 24/7 integrated situational awareness network, facilitating the gathering of public health intelligence and conducting daily risk assessments of potential public health risks/threats to Canadians.

Daily Risk Assessment

Shortly after the pandemic (H1N1) 2009, the Public Health Agency of Canada implemented a daily morning intelligence meeting to brief senior management of any perceived or real, current or potential threats to Canada or Canadians (at home and abroad) and to identify consequent actions. The approach considers all hazards: chemical, nuclear, biological, radiological, and environmental; natural or manmade; intentional and non-intentional. Examples include foodborne outbreaks, floods and hurricanes, emerging diseases, and bioterrorist activities.

This daily gathering of senior officials is more than a situational awareness briefing. It not only provides an overview of significant events occurring within Canada and globally, but is also a forum for discussion, assessment, decision-making, task delegation, and accountability. Participants at the meeting are engaged from across the various organizations of Canada's Health Portfolio: the Public Health Agency of Canada, Health Canada and the Canadian Food Inspection Agency. This facilitates efficient communication and awareness across the Portfolio, ensuring the engagement of all relevant sectors and strengthening Canada's capacity to rapidly identify risks and take the necessary actions.

Events brought forward at the daily meeting come in two types: official and unofficial reports. Official reports are generally brought forward by the areas within the Agency responsible for the content matter (referred to as program areas) in the form of confirmed case reports and outbreaks. Official reports also include IHR notifications as relayed through the IHR NFPO and other WHO and government communication identified by GPHIN. Unofficial reports are generally brought forward by GPHIN and distributed to the program areas for further assessment. These include media reports, journal publications, and Web postings synthesized by GPHIN analysts since the previous morning meeting.

Not all official and unofficial reports are discussed at the morning meeting. To facilitate the discussion, threats are assessed using the IHR-plus tool. However, reports do not have to necessarily meet a predefined set of criteria in order to be included for the morning meeting. This allows for an element of human judgment, and in the case of reports put forward by the GPHIN team, incorporates the analysts' historical, cultural and contextual knowledge and expertise.

The Broader Value of GPHIN

During a Public Health Event of Concern

The SARS outbreak introduced a new level of understanding about the utility and value of event-based surveillance systems. The GPHIN demonstrated its critical role in detecting the onset of an outbreak and throughout the progression of the event – as it was also capable of depicting evolution of the disease over time (Heymann 2010; WHO 2003). During the course of the outbreak, other related information was gleaned from the news media and other publicly available Websites for airlines, travel agencies, airports, as well as ministries of health, agriculture, and food safety. Concrete actions undertaken by states to curtail the threat posed by the outbreak in order to protect their citizens and economic interests were documented and disseminated in a timely manner. This resulted in the generation of reports on public health measures applied by countries, such as entry and exit screening at borders, quarantine and isolation practices, travel advisories, trade bans and travel cancellations. What is also worth noting is the way in which public health institutions, governments and international organizations were using news media to help manage the outbreak and also inform their risk communication strategy.

This was the beginning of a breakthrough where countries began to recognize the power of news media and other communication mediums (cell phones, blogs, etc.), and the need to be forthcoming in communicating in a timely manner about emerging public health threats that may have international implications.

While departments were trying to gather verified information, GPHIN was able to consolidate information from news media, industry and official websites about the spectrum of public health measures being considered or implemented by countries worldwide. This information was provided to stakeholders such as the Department of Foreign Affairs and helped inform the decision-makers responsible for managing the SARS outbreak.

This multidimensional approach towards the characterization of an event using open source data has since been repeated successfully during the avian influenza A(H5N1) outbreak and pandemic (H1N1) 2009. The information produced through this proven process has become an important component for decision-makers and is now an integral part of event – based surveillance at the agency.

During Mass Gathering Events

Mass gathering events (MGE) present opportunities for increasing the spread of communicable diseases or risk for intentional acts of terror. To minimize the risk of such threats, an enhanced surveillance strategy is necessary. The World Youth Day (WYD) held in Toronto, Canada, in 2002, drew an estimated 800,000 youths and was the largest single religious event in Canadian history (The Blade 2002). This event provided the opportunity for GPHIN to support the enhanced surveillance team that was assigned to this event. Activities entailed the monitoring, identification and daily reporting of situations such as demonstrations, adverse weather conditions, security at the event location, and infectious disease incidents occurring nationally and worldwide that may have implications for the WYD. The lessons learned from this MGE have now been applied to other MGEs occurring worldwide, including the 2007 World Cricket Cup, 2010 Winter Olympics, 2012 Festival of Pacific Arts, and 2012 Summer Olympics.

The GPHIN Difference

The GPHIN system is one among a limited suite of well-documented event-based surveillance systems (Keller et al. 2009; Hartley et al. 2010; Hartley et al. 2013). However, each system has its own strengths. In the case of the GPHIN system, it is the analysis and reporting enriched by the cadre of multidisciplinary, multicultural and multilingual human analysts.

The global security landscape is ever changing, fueled in part by failed states and conflicts that compromise or dismantle public health infrastructure. This weakens global health security and therefore requires constant vigilance by the GPHIN analysts to be able to detect any potential public health risk to the international community.

Sources feeding GPHIN are not only useful for the early detection of potential threats, but also for identifying response activities, such as public health measures implemented by countries. For example, GPHIN reports on trade bans were reviewed by the World Trade Organization (WTO) during the 2009 A(H1N1) pandemic for trade restricting and distorting measures (WTO 2009). This information proved to be useful for the WTO since their members, with the exception of four, neglected to notify them of any measures taken as a direct result of the outbreak.

IHR (2005) also urges the timely reporting of potential public health events of international concern within or outside the territory of the state party. To be able to meet this obligation requires not only the reliance on a state's national surveillance system, but also on other forms of surveillance that are capable of monitoring and providing near real – time information about all hazards that could constitute a potential public health risk of international concern. Event – based surveillance systems such as GPHIN have demonstrated the capacity to fill this void (Kumanan et al. 2008)

The results of the 2011 annual questionnaire designed by WHO Headquarters to monitor the progress being made in the implementation of the IHR and development of core capacities showed that State Parties were integrating event-based surveillance as part of their surveillance systems (WHO 2012a). A total of 161 out of 194 State Parties completed the 2011 questionnaire, and 96% of the Parties reported that they had designated units for event-based surveillance. This was a 9% increase from 2010.

Although State Parties may have designated units to conduct event-based surveillance, resources to support this activity may pose a challenge. GPHIN experience highlights the fact that having a tool that presents information about emerging public health situations is only the first step. The process for gleaning public health intelligence from these preliminary reports is the foundation that determines the effectiveness of using such a tool. This requires human analysis that cannot be replaced by a fully automated process.

Canada co-sponsored World Health Assembly Resolution 65.23, which calls for collaboration among State Parties, the WHO, and other relevant organizations and partners (WHO 2012b). As part of Canada's commitment, membership to GPHIN has been made available to member-states' national focal points to enhance their capacity to monitor public health events of international concern. Reports produced by GPHIN, such as those describing public health measures implemented worldwide during an event, help to inform decision makers. Since the implementation of public health measures is not in and of itself a reportable action by WHO member states under the IHRs, GPHIN reports are a significant complement to the overall monitoring of and response to the event.

The Road Ahead

When it was first conceived and built in 1997 as a prototype, GPHIN was ahead of its time, a pioneer in the field of public health, particularly event-based surveillance and early detection. Much has changed since then; certainly in terms of ever-evolving technology, but more importantly, in the way people use and share information. Traditional print media has become predominantly Web-based, with journalists steadily increasing their social media presence. For example, by the end of 2004, its first year in business, Facebook had a 'mere' one million users; by September 2012, it had surpassed the one billion user mark (Associated Press 2013). Other popular social media sites such as LinkedIn and Twitter have enjoyed similar success. Individuals and organizations continue to post more and more data online, with public health organizations actively participating in the social media space. For example, the Public Health Agency of Canada routinely tweets about seasonally relevant conditions, upcoming events, and emerging threats. Examples include Lyme disease and hantavirus in the summer; precautions for Hajj pilgrims following the identification of the Middle East Respiratory Syndrome Coronavirus (MERS-CoV); and travel health advisories.

The volume of data – whether it is pages and pages of online documents, user-loaded videos, or billions of short snippets of 140 characters or less – is now available to any individual with Internet access. This means that we are literally overcrowded with information. This 'big' volume of data from across countless sources is available with a few simple clicks; 'Big Data' is an understatement. However, though simple to access, analysis of the sheer volume and complex multidimensional nature of this data is another thing altogether.

As public health strives to keep up with these societal and technological drifts and shifts, new approaches and innovative thinking are required. The lines between traditional 'indicator-based surveillance' and nontraditional methods, such as event-based surveillance, have become blurred, with semantics providing a false dichotomy between the two. The solution, however, is not to necessarily make systems such as GPHIN 'one-stop' surveillance shops, but rather to build them into comprehensive public health surveillance activities. The daily meetings held within Canada's Health Portfolio are a step in this direction, integrating different sources of health data to provide intelligence. However, this approach is only the first step to comprehensive public health surveillance and intelligence, and the value of being able to synthesize information from multiple disciplines to identify signals of potential threats remains largely untapped. As the BioCaster example in Chapter 6 highlights, as methods for 'Big Data' visualization and analytics continue to evolve, organized public health must participate or risk becoming irrelevant to a data – hungry and rapidly shrinking globalized world.

While the complex challenges of 'Big Data' present invaluable opportunities, they also raise dangerous and unwanted ones. Advertising and marketing have become targeted based on browsing habits and online activity as individuals post opinions, pictures and stories implicating themselves and others. Issues of privacy and ethical online conduct have become frequent topics of discussion but to date, regulation remains largely a corporate and individual responsibility. As health is a very personal topic for many, public health initiatives must therefore be extremely sensitive to these issues, engaging the public in a way that respects their privacy but provides demonstrable value.

One way to achieve this is through crowd participation: crowdsourcing of information feeding into comprehensive public health surveillance activities. This may come from experts; for example, in addition to the value that GPHIN's human analysts bring, users of the GPHIN system are encouraged to provide feedback, commentary and content back to the program. It should be noted that while this aspect of the network does require formalization and strengthening, its value and importance are duly recognized. However, this may also come from members of the public, who may be just as inclined to report on their daily health status as they are on their relationship status, daily (sometimes hourly) activities and locations through social media. However the incorporation of information from the public raises a significant issue, inherent to 'Big Data' approaches: noise. Public health is intimately familiar with issues of sensitivity and specificity, and the challenge to remaining relevant is remaining valid and reliable. In turn, validity and reliability necessitate the development of appropriate evaluation metrics to determine the overall value and direction of development and implementation.

Conclusion

It is often said that in today's world, disease knows no borders, and we have seen countless examples of this. US President Obama clearly articulated this issue at the United Nations General Assembly in September 2011:

> To stop disease that spreads across borders, we must strengthen our system of public health ... we must come together to prevent, detect, and fight every kind of biological danger – whether it is a pandemic like H1N1, a terrorist threat, or a treatable disease. (Miller and Dowell 2012)

To be able to bolster the global health security and reduce the global disease burden inflicting on humanity, the global community will need to take leadership and action to resolve the global disparity between the rich and poor nations and the structural inequalities within the countries themselves (Aldis 2008; Bond 2008; Feldbaum et al. 2010). This includes addressing vaccine preventable diseases, potable drinking water, sanitary conditions and sustainable environments.

Similarly, data and information have become borderless, not only flowing freely around the globe, but also impossible to contain due to sheer breadth and volume. Public health would do well to capitalize on the evolution of technology and the social paradigm shifts that accompany it, and this includes an evolution of thought regarding public health surveillance.

The continued development and integration of systems such as GPHIN are paramount to this evolution and to the growing field of health security. However, the success of these initiatives in a borderless world requires borderless cooperation and communication, which in turn require appropriate governance to define expectations and measure progress.

We must therefore strive to continually work together to refine our surveillance systems, learning from the events, threats and disasters of the past to ensure our relevance in the present and secure our health and safety for generations to come.

References

Aldis, W. 2008. Health security as a public health concept: A critical analysis. *Health Policy and Planning*, 23: 369–73.

Associated Press 2013. *Number of active users at Facebook over the years*. [online] Available at: http://bigstory.ap.org/article/number-active-users-facebook-over-years-5 [Accessed: 8 November 2013].

Beaglehole, R. and Bonita, R. 2009. *Global Public Health: A New Era*, 2nd Edition. Oxford: Oxford University Press.

Bond, K. 2008. Health security or health diplomacy? Moving beyond semantic analysis to strengthen health systems and global cooperation. *Health Policy and Planning*, 23: 376–8.

Burns, W. 2006. Openness is key in fight against disease outbreaks. *Bulletin of the World Organization*, 84(10): 769–70.

Cash, R.A. and Narasimhan, V. 2000. Impediments to global surveillance of infectious diseases: Consequences of open reporting in a global economy. *Bulletin of the World Health Organization*, 78: 1358–67. Available at: http://www.who.int/bulletin /archives/78%2811%291358.pdf [Accessed: 9 November 2013].

Cerny P.G. 1993. Globalization and the changing logic of collective action. *International Organization*, 49(4): 595–625.

Davies, S.E. 2008. Securitizing infectious disease. *International Affairs*, 84(2): 295–313.

Davies, S.E. 2012. *Global Politics of Health*. Malden, MA: Polity Press.

Davies, S.E. and Youde, J. 2012. Special section: The politics of disease surveillance. *Global Change, Peace & Security*, 24(1): 53–6.

FAO, OIE and WHO. 2006. *Global Early Warning and Response System for Major Animal Disease, including Zoonoses (GLEWS)*. [online] Available at: http://www.oie.int/fileadmin/Home/eng/About_us/docs/pdf/GLEWS_Tripartite-Finalversion010206.pdf [Accessed: 9 November 2013].

Feldbaum, H., Lee, K. and Michaud, J. 2010. Global health and foreign policy. *Epidemiologic Review*, 32(1): 82–92.

Gill, S. and Law, D. 1988. *The Global Political Economy: Perspectives, Problems and Policies*. Baltimore, MD: The Johns Hopkins University Press.

Grein, T.W., Kamara, K.O., Rodier, G., et al. 2000. Rumors of disease in the global village: Outbreak verification. *Emerging Infectious Diseases*, 6(2): 97–102.

Hartley, D.M., Nelson, N.P., Walters, R., et al. 2010. Landscape of international event – based biosurveillance. *Emerging Health Threats Journal*, e3. Published online. doi:10.3134/ehtj.10.003

Hartley, D.M., Nelson, N.P., Arthur, R., et al. 2013. An overview of Internet biosurveillance. *Clinical Microbiology and Infection*, 19(11): 1006–13.

Health Canada 2006. *Health Canada's GOL Journey to Success*. [online] Available at: http://www.hc-sc.gc.ca/ahc-asc/pubs/_gol-idg/2006/index-eng. php [Accessed: 8 November 2013].

Heymann, D. 2010. Keynote lecture: Recognizing the next SARS and the role of surveillance. *Influenza and Other Respiratory Viruses*, 4(Suppl. 2): 3–9.

Heymann, D.L. and Rodier G.R. 2001. Hot spots in a wired world: WHO surveillance of emerging and re-emerging infectious diseases. *Lancet Infectious Diseases*, 1(5): 345–53.

Hitchcock, P., Chamberlain, A., Van Wagoner, M., et al. 2007. Challenges to global surveillance and response to infectious disease outbreaks of international importance. *Bisecurity and Bioterrorism: Biodefense Strategy, Practice, and Science*, 5(3): 206–27.

Keller, M., Blench, B., Tolentino, H. et al. 2009. Use of unstructured event – based reports for global infectious disease surveillance. *Emerging Infectious Disease*, 15(5): 689–95.

Korda, H. and Itani, Z. 2011. Harnessing social media for health promotion and behaviour change. *Health Promotion Practice*, 14(1): 15–23.

Kumanan, W., von Tigerstrom, B. and McDougall, C., 2008. Protecting global health security through the International Health Regulations: Requirements and challenges. *Canadian Medical Association Journal*, 179(1): 44–8.

Mawudeku, A., Blench, M., Boily, L., et al. 2013. The Global Public Health Intelligence Network, in *Infectious Disease Surveillance*, 2nd Edition (eds N.M. M'ikanatha, R. Lynfield, C.A. Van Beneden and H. de Valk), Oxford: John Wiley & Sons Ltd.

Miller, R. and Dowell, S.F. 2012. *Investing in a safer United States: What is global health security and why does it matter?* Center for Strategic and International Studies, Washington DC [online] Available at: http://csis.org/files/publication/120816_Miller_InvestingSaferUS_Web.pdf [Accessed: 9 November 2013].

Minister of Justice. 2006. *Public Health Agency of Canada Act*. [online] Available at: http://lois-laws.justice.gc.ca/PDF/P-29.5.pdf [Accessed: 9 November 2013].

Minister of Justice. 2007. *Emergency Management Act*. [online] Available at: http://lois-laws.justice.gc.ca/PDF/P-29.5.pdf [Accessed: 9 November 2013].

Mykhalovskiy, E. and Weir, L. 2006. The Global Public Health Intelligence Network and early warning outbreak detection: A Canadian contribution to global public health. *Canadian Journal of Public Health*, 97(1): 42–4.

National Advisory Committee on SARS and Public Health. 2003. *Learning from SARS – renewal of public health in Canada: A report of the national advisory committee on SARS and public health.* [online] Available at: http://www.phac-aspc.gc.ca/publicat/sars-sras/naylor/ [Accessed: 8 November 2013].

O'Brien, R. and Williams, M. 2013. *Global Political Economy: Evolution and Dynamics, 4th Edition.* New York, NY: Palgrave Macmillan.

Organization for Economic Co-Operation and Development 1996. *ICT Standardisation in the New Global Context: Final Report.* Paris. [online] Available at: http://www.oecd.org/sti/2094715.pdf [Accessed: 8 November 2013].

Paquet, C, Coulombier, D., Kaiser, R. et al. 2006. Epidemic intelligence: A new framework for strengthening disease surveillance in Europe. *Eurosurveillance*, 11(12): 665. [online] Available at: http://www.eurosurveillance.org/ViewArticle.aspx?ArticleId=665 [Accessed: 8 November 2013].

Public Safety Canada 2011. *An Emergency Management Framework for Canada.* 2nd Ed. [online] Available at: http://www.publicsafety.gc.ca/cnt/rsrcs/pblctns/mrgnc-mngmnt-frmwrk/index-eng.aspx#a01 [Accessed: 9 November 2013].

The Blade 2002. *Lifelong pilgrimage: World Youth Day's impact could linger.* 3 August 2002.

Tulchinsky, T.H. and Varavikova, E.A. 2009. *The New Public Health*, 2nd Edition. Burlington, MA: Academic Press, 6–19.

World Health Organization 2003. *The World Health Report 2003 – Shaping the Future.* [online] Available at: http://www.who.int/whr/2003/en/whr03_en.pdf [Accessed: 9 November 2013].

World Health Organization 2008a. *International Health Regulations (2005)*, 2nd Edition. [online] Available at: http://whqlibdoc.who.int/publications/2008/9789241580410_eng.pdf [accessed 8 November 2013].

World Health Organization 2008b. *Communicable disease alert and response for mass gatherings: Key considerations.* [online] Available at: http://www.who.int/csr/Mass_gatherings2.pdf [Accessed: 9 November 2013].

World Health Organization 2012a. *Summary of 2011 States Parties Report on IHR Core Capacity Implementation* [online] Available at: http://www.who.int/ihr/publications/WHO_HSE_GCR_2012.10_eng.pdf [Accessed: 9 November 2013].

World Health Organization 2012b. *Implementation of the International Health Regulations (2005).* 65th World Health Assembly, 2012 May 21–26; Geneva (Switzerland). Geneva: WHO; 2012 (Resolution WHA65.23) [online] Available at: WHA http://apps.who.int/gb/ebwha/pdf_files/WHA65/A65_R23-en.pdf [Accessed: 9 November 2013].

World Health Organization and Food and Agricultural Organization 2013. INFOSAN *Activity Report: 2011–2012.* Geneva: WHO Press. [online] Available at: http://www.fao.org/fileadmin/user_upload/agns/pdf/Infosan/INFOSAN_Activity_Report_2011-2012_-_Final.pdf [Accessed: 9 November 2013].

World Trade Organization 2009. *Report To The TPRB From The Director-General On The Financial And Economic Crisis And Trade-Related Developments.* WT/TPR/OV/W/2. [online] Available at: http://www.wto.org/english/news_e/news09_e/tpr_13jul09_dg_report_e.doc [Accessed: 9 November 2013].

Zacher, M.W. and Keefe, T.J. 2008. *The Politics Of Global Health Governance: United By Contagion.* New York, NY: Palgrave Macmillan.

Chapter 6
A Review of Web-based Epidemic Detection

Nigel H. Collier

Introduction

Epidemic intelligence (EI) is the early identification, assessment, and verification of potential public health hazards (Paquet et al. 2006) and the timely dissemination of alerts to appropriate stakeholders. The discipline includes both indicator surveillance techniques such as sentinel networks of physicians as well as event techniques that gather data from internet-based digital news media (Hartley et al. 2010) in addition to official sources such as World Health Organization (WHO) alerts. Event techniques in particular, with their emphasis on sifting through large volumes of dynamically changing unstructured data, lie at the intersection of public health and informatics. The technological discipline that has grown from this and similar interactions is called text mining (Hearst 1999). Text mining is a relatively new human language processing technology that aims to meet the knowledge discovery needs of professionals struggling under pressure of information overload, be it from the need to find facts and opinions on the Internet or making new discoveries in literature databases like PubMed's Medline (Swanson 1986). Text mining aims to discover novel information in a timely manner from large-scale text collections by developing high performance algorithms for sourcing and converting unstructured textual data to a machine understandable format and then filtering this according to the needs of its users. In later stages, text mining systems perform domain analysis (e.g. to determine topical details or identify aberrations from past norms) and deliver results in customized forms so that users can rapidly synthesize situations of interest (Feldman and Sanger 2006).

    Whilst dictionary-based search techniques certainly have their role to play, text mining usually goes far beyond keyword searching used by traditional search engines to find a needle with a particular color, weight, and length in the proverbial haystack. Uncovering documents on the topic of malaria, for example, is no guarantee that the information contained in them is relevant to discovering a new epidemic. What is needed is to condense the facts contained in the document into a fixed format—an event frame—that embodies all aspects of interest to the expert: Is there a case reported? What are the symptoms? How severe are they? Where and when did the event happen? By incorporating sophisticated knowledge models, text mining aims to understand the meaning—the semantics—of texts, albeit in a limited area of human expertise.

Whilst text mining has application in many real life scenarios as diverse as business intelligence, patent searching, and market surveying, this chapter will highlight its contribution to the alerting of public health hazards in the online media and briefly categorize the relevant methods and resources available. I conclude by discussing possible future trends and research issues.

Background

As shown by Hartley et al.'s (2010) survey paper, event-driven surveillance systems are now widely used by national and trans-national public health organizations such as the WHO, the Centers for Disease Control and Prevention (CDC), and the European Centre for Disease Prevention and Control (ECDC), Public Health Agency of Canada (PHAC), and many other agencies. In November 2002 at the start of the SARS epidemic, the GPHIN system (Mawudeku and Blench 2006, see also Chapter 5) at PHAC was among the earliest, along with the ProMED network (Madoff and Woddall 2005), to provide early warning of the impending near-pandemic starting in Guandong Province in Southern China. During the A(H1N1) influenza pandemic in 2009 a number of systems are credited with the timely discovery of early events including MedISys (Steinberger et al. 2008), Veratect (Wikipedia 2009), HealthMap (Brownstein et al. 2008), and BioCaster (Collier et al. 2008). Tools such as Riff from InSTEDD (Fuller 2010) were used to enhance decision support by integrating signals from virtual teams of experts with multiple streams of data from EI systems such as EpiSpider (Tolentino et al. 2007), SMS messages, and electronic medical records in OpenMRS. Additionally the MEDCollector system also aims to integrate multiple Web-based sources (Zamite et al. 2010). Of historical interest are two early systems: Proteus-Bio (Grishman et al. 2002) and MiTAP (Damianos et al. 2002).

Figure 6.1 illustrates the range of services available in the BioCaster EI system, produced by an international team based in Japan. As an example of the power of semantics driven text mining consider the following scenario. A public health expert is interested in finding out about a possible fatal case of person-to-person transmission of A(H5N1) in a family in Thailand. The expert who is in the field logs into a public Web portal on her smartphone and enters *A(H5N1)* as the search term along with *Thailand*, the date range of interest and requests only English language news articles. Internally the system recognizes that the first term is an English variant of an index term in its disease ontology (*highly pathogenic H5N1 avian influenza*). The search is performed over thousands of possible events stored in the database, but the results do not appear relevant to the expert's need. The system then offers the user the choice of searching using the disease symptoms. The user selects to search using symptoms such as *cough, high fever, pneumonia, acute respiratory distress*, and all their synonyms. This time, an article is found, but the report is already two weeks out of date and missing some vital pieces of

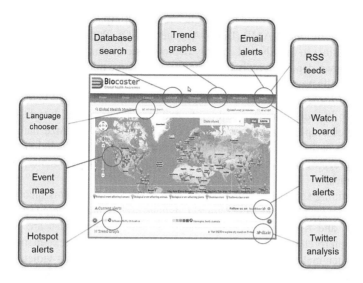

Figure 6.1   The BioCaster portal (http://born.nii.ac.jp) is a 24/7 system designed to deliver a variety of methods for enhanced access to epidemic events reported in news and social media

information about the name of the district and hospital. The user then chooses to search the Thai news, and the search is automatically repeated using Thai term equivalents. A structured table is produced summarizing each event in English with a flag indicating high priority items. The expert then finds the event that she is searching for and initiates a risk analysis procedure by transferring the event data to a secure watch board for sharing with colleagues. In summary, the key component in this system is the analyst herself, but the technology has enabled her to increase her productivity by rapidly gaining insight into the context of a cluster outbreak so she can help her colleagues make a more informed decision. The EI system has enabled her to supplement whatever indicator-based information sources might have been available to her and to communicate better with her human network of contacts. Though I do not claim that mining the Web for reports is the only viable solution to EI, it is possible that without this service the expert might initially have had to rely on word-of-mouth, circulated news clippings, or hit-and-miss ad hoc searches.

The scenario described above represents the high-end of automated EI systems but is feasible by fully applying today's technology. The availability of Web 2.0 services such as mapping (e.g. Google Maps [http://maps.google.com]/Bing Maps [http://www.bing.com/maps]), news aggregation (e.g. Google News [http://news. google.com]), photo sharing (e.g. Flickr [http://www.flickr.com]), video sharing (e.g. YouTube [http://www.youtube.com]), social media (e.g. Twitter [http://www. twitter.com]), text mining services (e.g. Open Calais [http://www.opencalais.

com]), and data converters (e.g. Google Translate [http://translate.google.com]) along with traditional LAMP (Linux-Apache-MySQL-Python) architectures has made it possible to rapidly and cheaply deploy systems that can ingest, filter, and visualize news data and individual reports posted on microblogging sites like Twitter. As illustrated in the example, high-end systems combine such generic services into so-called Web 2.0 *mashups* together with specialized knowledge of the domain in order to reduce ambiguity and increase precision. Interfaces often employ web-mapping services such as Google Maps to organize data simply across time and space. Users can then explore domain specific relations, drill down, aggregate across events, and communicate their findings and interpretations to colleagues.

Text mining services running on the back-end of such systems incorporate a rich fusion of technologies from natural language processing, machine translation, ontologies and reasoning. The challenges to these technologies are to make accurate interpretations of massive volumes of multilingual text in near real-time and then make judgments about whether the detected events violate domain norms. Seemingly innocuous contexts such as vaccination campaigns, bursts of media interest in politicians/pop idols such as *Obama Fever/Bieber Fever*, and vague reports of mystery illnesses are all challenge areas for automated text understanding. Trying to see through the fog of media interest to extrapolate case counts is also a challenging area complicated by the seeming lack of correlation with published news reports.

In the remainder of this chapter I will look in more detail at some of the issues surrounding text mining services which lie at the heart of semantic data extraction from free text at the same time as synthesizing my research in this area over the last six years.

Core Technologies

In this section I aim to give a broad impression of the automated technologies involved in text mining for EI. Events start with the biology in the real world and then through a process we still know too little about, media organizations report some of these events in digital form. From this point text mining systems have a chance to pick up the story in a trawl of the Web and convert the free text data into a structured event frame for sharing. The news story as a structured event frame is then analyzed using both statistics and human analysts. This might lead to the event being flagged as an immediate alert for verification, put on a watch list or archived for future reference.

While my focus is on automated methods, as the previous chapters have discussed, human users naturally have a vital role to play at many levels: (a) skilled human analysts perform risk analysis and verification; (b) the general public can help suggest or rate reports in a process called crowdsourcing, e.g. in HealthMap; and (c) users of social media sites can comment on their own health conditions on open access social media sites such as Twitter which can be aggregated for trend detection, e.g. in BioCaster's DIZIE project (Collier and Doan 2012a).

Data Sourcing

Whilst accurate statistics are hard to find, the World Wide Web (Web) is now one of the primary information sources for people seeking information (Janson and Spink 2006). Anyone with Web-browsing software has almost instant low-cost access to an extensive range of electronic news reports, blogs, search, and academic bulletins. EI systems can tap into this data in a variety of ways.

The lowest-cost option for computers to systematically work through this wealth of information is to harness a Web crawler. When pointed at a list of news sites this software will systematically trawl the links and download any pages that are new. Such an approach though incurs a hidden cost in the maintenance of software to decode the HTML template for each Web site so that informative content can be separated from non-relevant content such as metadata, adverts, images, headlines for other stories, and hyperlinks. Given the huge variety of templates and their constant revision the manual effort in maintaining such software is considerable. Several groups have developed generic content discovery algorithms based on heuristic rules and statistical models (e.g. Lin and Ho 2002) but ready to use software may be difficult to find in the public domain.

A more efficient approach to locating news is to use the power of RSS feeds—syndicated news provided in a structured XML format. This option allows EI systems to regularly poll news servers, pull out links to new stories and download their content. The issue of content discovery on the news page is still a problem though.

Although freely available, public news aggregators such as Google News and Yahoo News have access to a very wide range of sources, for mission critical systems as well as to ensure coverage several EI systems have contracts with private news aggregation companies such as Factiva and LexisNexis. These companies offer the widest possible range of sources across a variety of languages with clean content. A practical question for system builders is to ensure quality of geographic coverage. This is not always so simple to achieve given the inherent biases in each media source.

Text Analysis

Once news articles have been captured the first stage of semantic analysis is to filter them for topical relevancy. The techniques used here that have enjoyed the most success are usually data driven based either on supervised (Conway et al. 2009), semi-supervised (Torii et al. 2011) or unsupervised machine learning. These techniques are distinguished by how much use they make of pre-classified example data.

Text mining systems are designed around a clearly defined task specification such as a case definition like "Identify all infectious disease outbreak reports that contain evidence for human to human transmission" or "Identify all events consist with the International Health Regulation Annex 2 Decision Instrument."

To convert the unstructured data from a Web document into a structured event frame the computer requires knowledge about the syntactic and semantic structure of the language as well as the target output structure. This requirement tends to make text mining a language and domain-specific technology requiring interdisciplinary collaboration to develop system rulebooks. Building expert knowledge into a computer system for a specific task is economical only if the text collection is very large—such as the Web—and the nature of the information being found makes it very valuable to users. In addition to custom-built EI systems such as BioCaster, HealthMap, Epispider and MediSys, several private companies market generic text mining solutions including SAS, SPSS, Nstein and LexisNexis. Widely used open source toolkits include NLTK (http://nltk.org), the R project's text mining package (http://cran.r-project.org), and Sheffield University's GATE project (http://gate.ac.uk).

For computers to extract high quality information from text requires some degree of linguistic understanding. Systems typically require two sets of knowledge: domain knowledge that shows the classes of objects of interest and their relationships, and the patterns that show how these relationships are realized in the language of an actual text.

Most text mining systems start with a specialized module for recognizing the names of important entities in the text, a process called named entity recognition (NER) (Nadeau and Sekine 2007) that can be done using either data driven techniques such as support vector machines (SVMs) or rule-based techniques (see Table 6.1). I illustrate this with an example from the BioCaster system's rulebook which has the following pattern:

D21 :- name(disease) { list(%virus) "outbreak" }

In the language of SRL (Collier et al. 2010) this rule indexed as D21 identifies objects of type DISEASE. It states that a sequence of words should be labeled as a DISEASE type if it matches to an entry in the virus list and is followed by the string "outbreak." The output of this rule is to insert information into the text in the form of inline XML annotation for use in later processing steps. For example, the text "The AH1N1 outbreak occurred in communities across the region" would be recognized internally as "The <DISEASE>AH1N1 outbreak </DISEASE> occurred across the region." Following from NER is usually a stage of normalization so that surface forms of names get linked to a unique identifier in a dictionary or ontology, i.e. a structured conceptual representation of the terms and relationships in the domain.

Table 6.1   Summary of steps in text mining systems for epidemic intelligence

---

Data ingestion is usually the first stage with a variety of textual sources such as e-mails, homepages, Really Simple Syndication (RSS) feeds, Microsoft Office files and Portable Document Format (PDF) documents.

Data cleaning is vital in practice to remove unwanted noise from the text (such as advertisements or links to unrelated news stories) and to join together broken sentences. At this stage systems often try to break down large documents that talk about multiple topics into separate sections in a process called *Zoning* in order to remove noise or reclassify the document [24].

Data triage assigns the document a topic category for either trashing—in the case of non-relevant documents—or subsequent processing using detailed fact extraction. At this stage redundant information—multiple reports of the same event—are detected through document clustering. This stage is also intended to remove the most obvious true negatives but systems may struggle to handle the more subtle cases on the borderline of their task definitions leading to high numbers of false positives.

Fact extraction obtains structured information about an event such as the name of the disease, the type of agent, the number of victims and time and location where the event happened. With this information the computer can then begin to answer questions such as what happened, to who, where and when.

Ranking is done by applying rules on the results of earlier stages of processing. High-end systems will use sophisticated statistical analysis to assign an alerting level based on a comparison of aggregated data in the present and past. In practice, this is often the most difficult stage for systems to perform automatically with high levels of accuracy.

Human judgment is a key stage in the process. It is almost always needed to understand what is abnormal, to discovery rare events that the system may have missed, to make the final decision about vague reports and to link together disparate events. The limitations of the system will be most visible to the user at this stage and they have to apply their own judgments to correct for nuances of meaning that are clear to people but opaque to the computer software. Human analytical skills will also be able to discovery regularities in the data that can lead them to investigate new paths not available to current automated approaches.

In SRL more sophisticated rules can be made to identify relations consisting of one or more objects like DISEASE, VIRUS, PERSON, SYMPTOM, ORGANIZATION, LOCATION and so on. For example,

FW99: farm_worker("true") :- "death" "of" name*(person,P) { list(@farming_ occupation)}

Rule FW99 is another string matching rule that looks for sequences of words showing the death of farm workers. If the rule matches then it outputs "farm_ worker("true")," i.e. the left hand side of the ":-." The rule states that the string must match with a PERSON type containing a farming occupation listed in the dictionary such as abattoir workers, breeders, livestock handlers, veterinarians, ranchers etc. So for example, the text "The ministry announced the death of <PERSON>2 slaughterhouse workers</PERSON> from the virus" would successfully match this rule.

Whilst regular expression patterns like SRL can be quite effective, they are vulnerable to sensitivity constraints due to the large variety of surface patterns that need to be explicitly modeled. As in biomedical applications, more robust solutions are expected to come from full sentence parsing to uncover grammatical relations between words and phrases. Full parsing will also help to capture subtle aspects of the event such as polarity, certainty, and temporality that can be hard to capture using regular expressions. However, full parsing may come at a cost to computational efficiency and potentially create a bottleneck when timeliness is one key criterion for usability. This is particularly important during bursts of information that can occur during major epidemics.

Understanding time and location are key foundations for high quality EI (Chanlekha et al. 2010). In practice, though, there are many pitfalls. Document time stamps, for example, are not necessarily the best guide to decide on the time when a reported event took place. For example a document dated 2nd October 2008 might report "Last Tuesday avian influenza virus A was identified as the cause of an outbreak in two southern provinces of Viet Nam." We would expect the text mining system to record the date of the case as the 30th September 2008.

Additionally, location names are also often highly ambiguous in practice. For example, an equine influenza outbreak in Camden during the summer of 2007 would have to be identified as Camden near Sydney, Australia, and not as Camden in London, UK. Equally confusing for automated systems is the fact that an outbreak of Venezuelan hemorrhagic fever might not be taking place in Venezuela and an outbreak of a food-borne disease from eating satsumas would probably have no relation to Japan. Much research has taken place on identifying geo-political named entities such as countries and cities in general news texts (e.g. McCallum and Li 2003) with performance for English place names generally in the 80s to low 90s F-score on unseen texts, where F-score is the harmonic mean of recall and precision. Keller et al. (2009) provides a review of the issues for epidemic surveillance and presents a new method for tackling the identification of a disease outbreak location based on neural networks trained on surface feature patterns in a window around geo-entity expressions. The resulting 64% F-score appears at first sight to be lower than we might have expected. The performance gap may be due to the variety of contexts in which geographic expressions for disease outbreaks occur and the lack of training data available. Contextual information for deciding on whether one of many locations mentioned in a report is the actual disease outbreak location is often dependent on contextual clues outside the scope of a single sentence. For example, a local hospital may be mentioned as the place of treatment and the attributable source may be a health ministry spokesperson from the country's government. Since local names tend to be highly ambiguous both within and across countries, an EI system has a high chance of making a mistake in geo-coding the event based only on this first piece of information. It requires a combination of clues from the health ministry name and the local name to fix the actual specific location.

Because geo-temporal disambiguation is so difficult and because of the variety of ways in which cases are described across different news reports, it is challenging to completely de-duplicate news reports about events and obtain accurate tracking of case counts. One approach to do this is the spatio-temporal event calculus proposed by Chaudet (2006). Although the knowledge representation seems stable and repeatable, it is not clear yet how easily this can be operationalized.

Ontologies

It is clear that some *a priori* knowledge over and above that supplied in the media report is necessary for the text mining system to make sense of the report, e.g. to resolve sense ambiguities such as knowing that A(H1N1) influenza, swine flu, and swine flu A all refer to the same disease, understand idiomatic expressions such as Venezuelan Hemorrhagic Fever, and to exclude implausible contexts such as vaccination campaigns. Where does domain knowledge come from? Working systems often incorporate a fusion of knowledge both statistical and symbolic. For example, HealthMap's use of a neural network to detect the focus location of the outbreak is a statistical approach, and BioCaster's SRL rules for resolving the focus disease agent is a symbolic approach. Here I focus on the role of ontologies in EI that help automate human understanding of key concepts and relations to achieve the desired level of filtering accuracy.

One of the most important functions of ontologies is to decide how alike two concepts are to each other. Biomedical ontologies minimally contain lists of terms and their human definitions that are then given unique identifiers and arranged into classes with common properties. These classes are then structured according to principles of classification such as the subsumption ("is a") relation. For example, the Medical Subject Headings (MeSH) ontology (Lowe and Barnett 1994) says that the term "*influenza, human*" is a type of *respiratory tract infection*. Other widely known examples of ontologies for human understanding include SNOMED Clinical Terms (Price and Spackman 2000), the Foundation Model of Anatomy (Rosse and Mejino 2008), the Unified Medical Language System (UMLS) (Humphreys and Lindberg 1993: 170), and AGROVOC (Soergel et al. 2004). Community efforts such as the Open Biological and Biomedical Ontologies (2011) have come a long way in recent years towards forming standards for ontology construction, highlighting common pitfalls in their construction and promoting inter-operability.

In the domain of EI it is necessary to identify and link term classes such as DISEASE, SYMPTOM, and SPECIES in order to separate reports about human, animal or crop diseases. We might also include a CHEMICAL class if knowledge of chemical or nucleotide agents were important. In order capture geospatial reference we also need to define types for COUNTRY, PROVINCE, and

CITY. This would help to integrate information from the system with geospatial browsers such as Google Maps or NASA's World Wind.

Currently, there are few dedicated publicly available ontologies that contain all the terms necessary for EI systems. In addition to the general purpose biomedical ontologies mentioned above the commercial knowledge management tools Gideon (http://www.gideononline.com) has extensive coverage, contains a sophisticated reasoning engine and is widely used to support expert diagnosis but is closed source and not designed to interoperate with automated text analytics. Within open source resources, we have provided the BioCaster ontology (BCO) version 3 (Collier et al. 2010) in the OWL Semantic Web language to support automated reasoning across technical and laymen's terms in 12 languages for 336 conditions. The BCO supports a variety of relation types including term equivalence across languages, preferred term, causality between agents and conditions and between agents and symptoms. For example, if we find that a news document contains the disease "chicken pox" then the ontology informs the system that the causal agent is the "varicella-zoster virus," or if the news article mentions a disease outbreak of "swine flu" and another of "swine influenza A" then the ontology can provide a unifying root term of "A(H1N1) influenza." Another application for the ontology is in helping to choose appropriate levels of generality for disease names, for example if the document mentions both "highly pathogenic H5N1 avian influenza" and "avian influenza" then the event will be designated as the more specific of the two. In addition to human diseases it also covers animal diseases where the disease is a potential zoonotic threat to humans or can have severe economic consequences for society.

As a final note it is important to consider how to keep the ontology up-to-date. Although disease vocabulary is relatively stable, when new types of diseases strike such as "swine flu" during 2009, the nomenclature can evolve surprisingly rapidly. In the future we would like to explore community efforts (i.e. social media) to harness expertise for solving this issue.

Machine Translation

Given the very large volumes of media reports and the variety of human languages in which they are written, high throughput machine translation (MT) is usually required in order to make sense of news events in the timeliest manner (Wilks 2009). MT systems have been in widespread use for many years, e.g. the Systran system used by the European Commission, or Yahoo!'s Babelfish used for Web page translation. The fidelity of machine translation output generally varies from high for cognate language pairs such as English-French to mediocre for non-cognate pairs such as English-Japanese or English-Arabic. One issue complicating the choice of MT system is that it is not clear yet how quality of output impacts on the final performance of the EI system although we have seen in our own evaluations that MT output has proven useful for improving the timeliness and sensitivity of alerting (Eysenbach 2002; Collier 2011: S10).

A variety of general-purpose MT systems exist from commercial companies such as Google Translate or Microsoft's Bing Translate each allowing a wide range of language pairs at a cost that is typically based on the volume of text translated per month. Systems that can be installed and run on a local server such as the commercial Systran or the freely available MOSES have at least one advantage over general purpose MT systems which is that they can usually be customized to the domain vocabulary if sufficient quantities of example texts exist in both the source and target languages.

MT is often employed before text analysis, translating all languages to a common target language such as English so that rulebooks don't need to be developed and maintained for each language. MT is also useful to help analysts make a first pass at understanding the topicality and significance of news reports. However in the absence of fully automated high quality MT, end users will need access to bilingual analysts who can interpret the content and context of the source language directly.

Aberration Detection

Being able to detect a news report about a public health event is not enough to make an EI system useful. In order to have value EI systems must be able to differentiate between mundane and unusual reports in a timely manner and supply this information to people who can initiate the appropriate actions. Such systems must be flexible to adapt themselves to changing patterns of diseases without any bias for a particular country or language. In practice, human experts with familiarity of the country concerned will almost always be necessary to analyze and interpret warning signals. The question for text mining researchers and users is how far can the technology be trusted to detect aberrations and what kind of aberrations are capable of automated analysis? Given that the state of the physical world with regard to disease incidence is always changing and that new pathogens are constantly evolving this is not a problem that can be tackled solely using the static ontologies I discussed earlier.

Detecting aberrations relies on identifying metrics that strongly correlate to the target objectives of the system designers—the discipline of infodemiology that was coined by Eysenbach (2002). News reports push the limits of what can be achieved using early warning data because of their biases, inaccuracies and vagueness. For example, the data can be strongly driven by fear and socio-economic biases which need to be compensated for. In addition to natural language processing, making sense of underlying trends draws on several established empirical disciplines: (a) knowledge discovery in databases (Fayyad et al. 1996); and (b) time series analysis (Wagner et al. 2001; Buckeridge et al. 2005) for change point detection. Many algorithms exist in both areas that can be adapted to the task at hand and compared.

The first stage in modeling begins by deciding on the objectives of the system such as coverage, alerting speed, or low false alarm rates. A set of features are then identified, such as the name of the disease and the country or province where it occurred, before establishing strong temporal and spatial baselines based on aggregated counts of these features over a history period. Deviation from such baselines by a significant margin constitutes an alert. Deciding on how to calculate the baseline and deviation, e.g. using statistical process control methods, is an ongoing research topic (Buckeridge et al. 2005).

My previous work in BioCaster has looked at flagging aberrations for a broad range of diseases using features from the structured event frame, specifically the disease and country where the event took place. By using aggregated counts of news events I was able to obtain high levels of alerting performance on a range of diseases and outbreak sizes against ProMED as the silver standard baseline. I could also compare a range of models and feature types. Since the actual state of the physical world is not usually known, I considered ProMED's human moderated network to be a reasonable standard for event alerting. My comparisons of English and multilingual news (Collier 2010: 2011) showed high levels of performance for the CDC's Early Aberration and Reporting System's (EARS) C2 and C3 models (Hutwagner et al. 2003) with a 7-day baseline and 2-day buffer period. Both algorithms showed a good balance of F-score, timeliness, and false alarm rates.

A different approach is adopted by Von Etter et al. (2010) who use supervised classification on textual features using naïve Bayes and support vector machines to categorize outbreak events on a 0 to 5 scale of relevance (F-score 79.24% on SVM with an RBF-kernel).

Dissemination

Notifying alerts to users and other systems is the final key stage. At the present time no interoperable standard for message structure, semantics or vocabulary appears to have been agreed internationally among Web-based EI systems. Although standards such as the Common Alerting Protocol have been proposed, the most popular format currently in use may be GeoRSS, a lightweight XML format for syndicating links to Web content that encodes geographic information. Minimal necessary elements might include, for example, a unique message identifier, the time of the message, the time of the event, a uniformly agreed name for the disease, the outbreak location, the species affected, a description of the reporting source, the degree of certainty, the level of confidentiality of the report, the status of the report (e.g. a trial exercise), message type (e.g. an update or an error notification), and a unique identifier for the event by the reporting system.

Case Study: BioCaster

Background

BioCaster is a fully automated experimental system for near real-time 24/7 global health intelligence based at the National Institute of Informatics in Tokyo. Major goals of the research are: (a) to explore advanced algorithms for the semantic annotation of documents; (b) to acquire knowledge which can empower human language technologies; and (c) to investigate early alerting methods from news and open access social media signals. Analysis and validation of signals is assumed to take place downstream of the system by the community of users.

The concept of BioCaster (Collier et al. 2008) began in 2006 when grant-in-aid funding from the Japan Society for the Promotion of Science enabled the construction of a core high performance system (Collier et al. 2007) for semantic indexing of news related to disease outbreaks. At the start BioCaster's focus was on Asia-Pacific languages due to the perceived risk of newly emerging and re-emerging health threats in the region (Jones et al. 2008) such as highly pathogenic A(H5N1) influenza. Work therefore began in 2006 on the construction of a multilingual ontology (Collier et al. 2006) that would form the conceptual framework for the system—a freely available community resource containing a structured public health vocabulary.

The core team involved in BioCaster's development at the National Institute of Informatics is usually 3 or 4 members with expertise in computational linguistics and software engineering. In 2006, collaboration with a network of academic partners was quickly established including groups at the National Institute of Infectious Diseases (Japan), Okayama University (Japan), the National Institute of Genetics (NIG, Japan), Kasetsart University (Thailand), and the Vietnam National University (VNU, Vietnam). These groups provide expertise in software engineering, public health, genetics, and computational linguistics across several languages. Since 2007, BioCaster has partnered with the Early Alerting and Reporting Project of the Global Health Security Action Group, a G7 + Mexico + EC + WHO initiative bringing together stakeholders, EI experts, and system owners to share expertise and develop a common Web-based platform.

Funding

BioCaster is a non-governmental system developed with grant-in-aid support from national funding organizations. In 2009 BioCaster was awarded a 3-year grant-in-aid by the Japan Science and Technology (JST) Agency under the Sakigake program to investigate enhanced health threat understanding by computers.

Output

BioCaster's implicitly intended users are analysts working at national and international public health agencies but there has also been considerable interest from physicians, veterinarians, researchers and the general public. Unique user numbers tend to be in the thousands per month but can rise substantially during major epidemics such as pandemic A(H1N1) and cholera in Haiti. As shown in Figure 6.1 BioCaster makes its output available in several formats such as Google maps, graphs, GeoRSS feeds and email alerts. The Web portal operates in two modes: (1) a freely accessible mapping and graphing interface called the Global Health Monitor (see Figure 6.1); (2) a password restricted alerting interface which is currently used by a small test community of public and animal health experts. Additionally the open access multilingual ontology provides structured term sets in 12 languages and has been downloaded by over 250 academic, industrial and public health groups worldwide including the WHO.

Coverage

On a typical day BioCaster processes 30,000 reports. Of these, approximately 55% will be in English, 11% in Chinese (Mandarin), 7% in German, 7% in Russian, 6% in Korean, 5% in French, 3% in Vietnamese, 2% in Portuguese, 2% in Chinese (Cantonese) and the remainder in Thai, Italian, and Arabic. Approximately 200 reports will be considered relevant after full analysis has taken place. Eighty percent of these reports will pertain to human cases and the remainder to animals with a very small number of plant diseases.

The range of health threats in BioCaster were prioritized according to notifiable diseases at health ministries in major countries in the Asia-Pacific region, Europe, and North America as well as discussions with veterinarian and chemical, biological, radiological, and nuclear (CBRN) experts. In October 2011 the BioCaster database (GENI-DB) (Collier 2011) contained news event records (without personal identifiers) for over 176 infectious diseases and chemicals whilst the rulebook has the potential to find 182 human diseases, 143 zoonotic disease, 46 animal diseases, and 21 plant diseases. Additionally, 40 chemicals and 9 radio-nucleotides are also under surveillance.

Signals

In addition to direct signals on 18 concept types such as DISEASE, VIRUS, BACTERIUM, SYMPTOM, and LOCATION names, BioCaster also looks for various event features such as international travel, drug resistance as well as a number of STEEP (Social Technological Economic Environmental Political) indicators. These include school closures, shortages of vaccines and panic buying of commodities.

Data Sources

Data is ingested on a 1-hour cycle from with approximately 27,000 news items analyzed per day from news sources at a commercial news aggregation company, Google News, as well as various NPO and official sources such as WHO, OIE and European Media Monitor alerts. Additionally, BioCaster's sister project in social media analysis (DIZIE) is analyzing syndromic signals from the Twitter microblogging service. After testing is completed we expect to integrate DIZIE alerts within BioCaster.

User Feedback

BioCaster has been used by a variety of public health organizations including the European Centers for Disease Control (ECDC), the U.S. Centers for Disease Control and Prevention (CDC), and the Ministry of Health in Japan. User feedback has been encouraging both about the quality of information the system provided and its scope. Public health analysts have asked for us to customize the system to monitor mass gathering events such as the Shanghai Expo in 2010 or the London Olympics in 2012 as well as possible outcomes of environmental disasters such as the Gulf of Mexico oil spill in 2010. Animal health analysts have begun to see the potential for systems like BioCaster and have asked us to expand the range of diseases we monitor to include notifiable conditions for animals.

The area where BioCaster receives the most requests is in user interface. In 2006, we focused information on a global bio-geographic map. As BioCaster's coverage has increased we have found that the map can easily overwhelm users and an adaptable alerting system was needed. In 2010, we therefore introduced hotspot alerts to draw the user's attention to specific reports. However, there is still much to be done, such as removing duplication, clustering related events, and integrating reports across languages and media types.

The information we provide is inevitably biased by BioCaster's input sources that rely heavily on Google News. In recent years, we have expanded BioCaster's language coverage to include news in several other languages such as Spanish, Vietnamese, and Chinese, but the source engine still appears to have a US-centric focus with significant gaps for sub-Saharan Africa and parts of middle-Asia. We are currently trying to supplement the system with other sources such as news aggregators in China. In a seminal study of epidemic intelligence systems, a recent study by Lyon et al. (2011) compared BioCaster, HealthMap, and Epispider over the period from 2nd to 30th August 2010 and found similar timeliness between the system alerts as well as complementarities in geographical and language focus between all three systems. The report highlighted the issue of automated location detection, e.g. BioCaster's missing of Pakistan during the study period. We have since corrected this anomaly but in the process discovered a number of issues stemming from the transliteration into English of place names in certain locations.

Future Developments

Our current work on aberration detection has touched upon only the explicitly stated facts in news media reports. More sophisticated text mining techniques hold out the potential for greater accuracy. For example, using multivariate features such as STEEP indicators, or symptom severity features might help to piece together seemingly disparate facts in order to better understand the significance of rare events. An improved model for spatial dispersion of events would also help. For example, a report of a mystery illness in two villages in northeastern Italy might not in itself be significant enough to trigger an alert. However the report could take on more significance if it were combined with the facts that: (a) there were an unusually high number of cases; (b) several victims complained of mild to severe joint pain and severe headache; (c) the first cases included a traveler from Kerala, India; (d) there had been a recent severe outbreak of Chikungunya in Kerala; and (e) the health authorities were recommending precautions to prevent contact with mosquitoes and suspended all blood donations.

As a first measure, coarse grained granularity of time and location needs to be improved so that events can be pinpointed down to at least a city and a day of occurrence, reducing the "late warning" issue that I have noted elsewhere (Collier 2010), where the tail of news reports about past events gets confused with newer events that share the same geographic feature.

On the issue of evaluation, other domains of text mining such as literature mining for bioinformatics (Hirschman et al. 2002) have made enormous progress in assessing quality, expanding participation, and improving performance by organizing shared evaluation challenges. In evaluations such as the DARPA sponsored TREC, TIPSTER, and MUC, systems are compared against a common task-based benchmark, allowing for both technical comparisons as well as user-based evaluation. However, adequate care needs to be taken to avoid "inbreeding" of participating systems through over-sharing of methods and resources. In contrast, in Web-based EI there has been relatively little community organization around evaluation or the sharing of tools and data. One recent study by Vaillant et al. (2011) shows progress in this area by comparing 7 EI systems for CBRN threats with a focus on sensitivity evaluation from a French public health perspective. Vaillant et al. show that by combining data from at least 4 systems over 94% sensitivity can be achieved. This result corroborates an earlier extrinsic evaluation highlighting high sensitivity and high timeliness perceived by users including international EI experts (2011). Further evaluation by the authors based on specific early warning indicators is still ongoing (personal communication) to assess event-based EI tools in a global public health context.

So far, I have implicitly assumed that digital news reports should be the main source of information for EI systems. In reality the landscape of digital sources is much richer: search queries, micro-blogs, digital radio, discussion boards, images, livecasts etc. Several works have already appeared looking at the potential to make use of individual health reports in Twitter (Signorini et al. 2011: e19467,

Lampos and Cristianini 2010: 411, 416; Doan and Collier 2012; Corley et al. 2010; Culotta 2010) for tracking influenza like illness. Pearson correlations with CDC surveillance reports from sentinel providers and UK GP reports have been very encouraging. Although microblogs have no editorial control, they contain a direct real-time view into the health conditions of individuals. Another source that has received attention are search engine query trends from Google and Yahoo! (Ginsberg et al. 2008; Polgreen et al. 2008). As with all short message sources, the challenge here is to interpret the search query's context; a user may query about a particular drug or health condition for a variety of reasons, e.g. general interest, a school report or concern about a health condition. Ginsberg's study clearly showed the potential to closely correlate query counts with CDC influenza data but research questions remain, particularly about geographic coverage as well as coverage across particular age groups, e.g. the young or old who may not be familiar or have access to the Internet. Other sources such as digital radio (potentially useful for countries in parts of Africa), SMS messaging, and livecast reports have yet to be explored.

The need for high performance computing to process data in real-time and adjust to surges during pandemics is a practical barrier to entry. Future systems may develop based around cloud computing services that are becoming available from companies such as Amazon, Google, and Microsoft.

Conclusion

In this chapter, I have uncovered only the surface of the complex technical aspects that Web-based EI system developers have grappled with over the last decade. Future developments in text mining will undoubtedly be necessary to harness the increasingly massive volumes of media and social network data and to combine this with non-media sources. There will also be constant challenges pertaining to the bias and geographic availability of data that covers all continents, as we have already seen in the cases of H1N1 (Chapter 2) and H5N1 (Chapter 8).

References

Berry, M.W. and Kogan, M. 2010. *Text Mining: Applications and Theory*. Chichester, UK: Wiley.

Brownstein, J.S., Freifeld, C.C., Reis, B.Y. and Mandl, K.D. 2008. Surveillance Sans Frontières: Internet-Based Emerging Infectious Disease Intelligence and the HealthMap Project. *Public Library of Science Medicine*, 5 (7), 1019–24.

Buckeridge, D., Burkom, H., Campbell, M., et al. 2005. "Algorithms for Rapid Outbreak Detection: A Research Synthesis. *Journal of Biomedical Informatics*, 38 (2), 99–113.

Chanlekha, H., Kawazoe, A. and Collier, N. 2010. A Framework for Enhancing Spatial and Temporal Granularity in Report-based Health Surveillance Systems. *BMC Medical Informatics and Decision Making*, 10 (1), 1–15.

Chaudet, H. 2006. Extending the Event Calculus for Tracking Epidemic Spread. *Artificial Intelligence in Medicine*, 38 (2), 137–56.

Collier, N. 2010. What's Unusual in Online Disease Outbreak News? *Journal of Biomedical Semantics*, 1 (2), 1–18.

_____. 2011. Towards Cross-lingual Alerting for Bursty Epidemic Events. *Journal of Biomedical Semantics*, 2 (5), s10–21.

Collier, N. and Doan, S. 2012a. Syndromic Classification of Twitter Messages. *Lecture Notes of the Institute for Computer Sciences, Social Informatics and Telecommunications Engineering*, 91, 186–95.

_____. 2012b. GENI-DB: A Database of Global Events for Epidemic Intelligence. *Bioinformatics*, 28 (8), 1186–8.

Collier, N., Kawazoe, A., Jin, L., et al. 2006. A Multilingual Ontology for Infectious Disease Surveillance: Rationale, Design and Challenges. *Language Resources and Evaluation*, 40 (3–4), 405–13.

Collier, N., Kawazoe, A., Shigematsu, M., et al. 2007. *Ontology-driven Influenza Surveillance from Web Rumours: Proceedings of the International Conference on Options for the Control Influenza VI* (Toronto: International Medical Press).

Collier, N., Doan, S., Kawazoe, A., et al. 2008. BioCaster: Detecting Public Health Rumors with a Web-based Text Mining System. *Bioinformatics*, 24 (24), 2940–41.

Collier, N., Goodwin, R.M., McCrae, J., et al. 2010. *An Ontology-driven System for Detecting Global Health Events*. Proceedings of the 23rd International Conference on Computational Linguistics, Beijing, China, 23–27 August, available at: http://aclweb.org/anthology/C/C10/C10-1025.pdf [Accessed: 12 October 2012].

Conway, M., Doan, S., Kawazoe, A. and Collier, N. 2009. Classifying Disease Outbreak Reports Using N-grams and Semantic Features. *International Journal of Medical Informatics*, 78 (12): e47–e58.

Corley, C.D., Cook, D.J., Mikler, A.R. and Singh, K.P. 2010. Text and Structure Data Mining of Influenza Mentions in Web and Social Media. *International Journal of Environmental Research and Public Health*, 7 (2), 596–615.

Culotta, A. 2010. *Detecting Influenza Outbreaks by Analyzing Twitter Messages: Proceedings of the First Workshop on Social Media Analytics*. New York: ACM.

Damianos, L., Ponte, J., Wohlever, S., et al. 2002. "MiTAP for Bio-security: A Case Study. *AI Magazine*, 23 (4), 13–29.

Doan, S. and Collier, N. 2012. Tracking the Influenza-like Illness (ILI) Rate by Analysing Twitter Data. *PLoS One* (under review).

Eysenbach, G. 2002. Infodemiology: The Epidemiology of (Mis)Information. *American Journal of Medicine*, 113, 763–5.

Fayyad, U., Piatetsky-Shapiro, G. and Smyth, P. 1996. From Data Mining to Knowledge Discovery in Databases. *AI Magazine*, 17 (3), 37–54.

Feldman, R. and Sanger, J. 2006. *The Text Mining Handbook: Advanced Approaches in Analyzing Unstructured Data.* Cambridge: Cambridge University Press.

Fuller, S. 2010. Tracking the Global Express: New Tools Addressing Disease Threats Across the World. *Epidemiology*, 21 (6), 769–71.

Ginsberg, J., Mohebbi, M., Patel, R., et al. 2008. Detecting Influenza Epidemics Using Search Engine Query Data. *Nature*, 457, 1012–14.

Grishman, R., Huttunen, S. and Yangarber, R. 2002. Information Extraction for Enhanced Access to Disease Outbreak Reports. *Journal of Biomedical Informatics*, 35 (4), 236–46.

Hartley, D., Nelson, N., Walters, R., et al. 2010. Landscape of International Event-based Biosurveillance. *Emerging Health Threats Journal*, 3 (3), 1–7.

Hearst, M. 1999. *Untangling Text Data Mining: Proceedings of the 37th Annual Meeting of the Association for Computational Linguistics.* College Park, MD: University of Maryland.

Hirschman, L., Park, J.C., Tsujii, J., et al. 2002. Accomplishments and Challenges in Literature Data Mining for Biology. *Bioinformatics*, 18 (12), 1553–61.

Humphreys, B. and Lindberg, D. 1993. The UMLS Project: Making the Conceptual Connection Between Users and the Information They Need. *Bulletin of the Medical Library Association*, 81 (2), 170–77.

Hutwagner, L., Thompson, W., Seeman, M.G. and Treadwell, T. 2003. The Bioterrorism Preparedness and Response Early Aberration and Reporting System (EARS). *Journal of Urban Health*, 80 (1), i89–96.

Janson, B. and Spink, A. 2006. How are we Searching the World Wide Web? A Comparison of Nine Search Engine Transaction Logs. *Information Processing and Management*, 42 (1), 248–63.

Jones, E., Patel, N., Levy, M., et al. 2008. Global Trends in Emerging Infectious Diseases. *Nature*, 451, 990–93.

Keller, M., Freifeld, C.C. and Brownstein, J.S. 2009. Automated Vocabulary Discovery for Geo-parsing Online Epidemic Intelligence. *BMC Bioinformatics*, 10 (385), 1–9.

Kosala, R. and Blockeel, H. 2000. Web Mining Research: A Survey. *SIGKDD Explorations*, 2 (1), 1–15.

Lampos, V. and Cristianini, N. 2010. *Tracking the Flu Pandemic by Monitoring the Social Web*, 2nd International Workshop on Cognitive Information Processing, Bristol, United Kingdom, 14–16 June 2010, Available at: http://ieeexplore.ieee.org/xpls/abs_all.jsp?arnumber=5604088&tag=1 [Accessed: 15 October 2012].

Lin, S. and Ho, J. 2002. *Discovering Informative Content Blocks from Web Documents*, Proceedings of ACM International Conference on Knowledge Discovery and Data Mining, Edmonton, Canada, 23–26 July. Available at: http://citeseerx.ist.psu.edu/viewdoc/summary?doi=10.1.1.18.7133 [Accessed: 12 October 2012].

Lowe, H. and Barnett, G. 1994. Understanding and Using the Medical Subject Headings (MeSH) Vocabulary to Perform Literature Searches. *Journal of the American Medical Association*, 271 (14), 1103–8.

Lyon, A., Nunn, M., Grossel, G. and Burgman, M. 2011. Comparison of Web-based Biosecurity Intelligence Systems: BioCaster, EpiSPIDER and HealthMap. *Tranboundary and Emerging Diseases*, 59 (3), 223–32.

Madoff, L.C. and Woodall, J.P. 2005. The Internet and the global monitoring of emerging diseases: Lessons from the first 10 years of ProMED. *Archives of Medical Research*, 36 (6), 724–30.

Mawudeku, A. and Blench, M. 2006. *Global Public Health Intelligence Network (GPHIN)*, 7th AMTA Conference, Cambridge, Massachusetts, August 8–12 2006, available at: http://www.mt-archive.info/MTS-2005-Mawudeku.pdf [Accessed: 11 October 2011].

McCallum, A. and Li, W. 2003. *Early Results for Named Entity Recognition with Conditional Random Fields, Feature Induction and Web-enhanced Lexicons.* Proceedings of the Seventh Conference on Natural Language Learning, Edmonton, Canada, 27 May to 1 June, available at: http://citeseerx.ist.psu.edu/viewdoc/download;jsessionid=3B11085DC43E272FCF8CB1377AE15196?doi=10.1.1.14.7963&rep=rep1&type=pdf [Accessed: 10 October 2012].

Nadeau, D. and Sekine, S. 2007. A Survey of Named Entity Recognition and Classification. *Linguisticae Investigationes*, 30 (1), 3–26.

Paquet, C., Coulombier, D., Kaiser, R. and Ciotti, M. 2006. Epidemic Intelligence: A New Framework for Strengthening Disease Intelligence in Europe. *EuroSurveillance*, 11 (12), 212–14.

Polgreen, P.M., Chen, Y., Pennock, D.M. and Nelson, F.D. 2008. Using Internet Searches for Influenza Surveillance. *Clinical Infectious Diseases*, 47 (11), 1443–8.

Price, C. and Spackman, K. 2000. SNOMED Clinical Terms. *British Journal of Healthcare Computing & Information Management*, 17 (3): 27–31.

Rosse, C. and Mejino, J.L.V. 2008. The Foundational Model of Anatomy Ontology, in *Anatomy Ontologies for Bioinformatics: Principles and Practice*, edited by A. Burger, D. Davidson and R. Baldock. London: Springer, 59–118.

Signorini, A., Segre, A.M. and Polgreen, P.M. 2011. The Use of Twitter to Track Levels of Disease Activity and Public Concern in the U.S. During the Influenza A H1N1 Pandemic. *PLoS One*, 6 (5): e19467.

Soergel, D., Lauser, B., Liang, A., et al. 2004. Reengineering Thesauri for New Applications: The AGROVOC Example. *Journal of Digital Information*, 4 (4), np.

Steinberger, R., Flavio, F., van der Goot, E., et al. 2008. Text Mining from the Web for Medical Intelligence, in *Mining Massive Data Sets for Security*, edited by F. Fogelman-Soulié et al. Amsterdam: IOS Press, 295–310.

Swanson, D.R. 1986. Fish Oil, Raynaud's Syndrome, and Undiscovered Public Knowledge. *Perspectives in Biology and Medicine*, 30(1), 7–18.

The Open Biological and Biomedical Ontologies. 2011. Available at: http://www.obofoundry.org/ [Accessed: 1 September 2011].

Tolentino, H., Kamadjeu, R., Fontelo, P., et al. 2007. Scanning the Emerging Infectious Disease Horizon—Visualizing ProMED Emails Using EpiSpider. *Advances in Disease Surveillance*, 2, 169.

Torii, M., Yin, L., Nguyen, T., et al. 2011. An Exploratory Study of a Text Classification Framework for Internet-based Surveillance of Emerging Epidemics. *International Journal of Medical Informatics*, 80 (1), 56–66.

Vaillant, L., Nys, J., Gastellu-Etchegorry, M. and Barboza, P. 2011. *Enhancement of Sensitivity with Gathering Internet-based Systems for Early Threat Detection within the Global Health Security Initiative (GHSI): The EAR Project: Proceedings of eHealth* (Malaga, Spain: EAR-GHSAG Group).

Vaillant, L., Barboza, P. and Arthur, R.R. 2011. *Epidemic Intelligence: Assessing Event-based Tools and User's Perception in the GHSAG Community: Proceedings of the International Meeting on Emerging Diseases and Surveillance* (Vienna: ProMED).

von Etter, P., Huttunen, S., Vihavainen, A., et al. 2010. *Assessment of Utility in Web Mining for the Domain of Public Health: Proceedings of NAACL HLT 2010 Workshop on Text and Data Mining of Health Documents* (Los Angeles, CA: NAACL).

Wagner, M.M., Tsui, F.C., Espino, J.U., et al. 2001. The Emerging Science of Very Early Detection of Disease Outbreak. *Journal of Public Health Management Practices*, 7 (6), 51–9.

Wikipedia 2009. *2009 Flu Pandemic Timeline*. Available at: http://en.wikipedia. org/wiki/2009_flu_pandemic_timeline [Accessed: 1 September 2011].

Wilks, Y. 2009. *Machine Translation—Its Scope and Limits*. London: Springer.

Zamite, J., Silva, F., Couto, F. and Silva, M. 2010. MEDCollector: Multisource Epidemic Data Collector. *Lecture Notes in Computer Science*, 6990, 40–72.

Chapter 7

GPHIN, GOARN, GONE? The Role of the World Health Organization in Global Disease Surveillance and Response

Clare Wenham

Introduction

Before the revised version of the International Health Regulations (IHR) went into effect in 2007, international disease surveillance and response was managed solely through the World Health Organization (WHO) and its member-states. Any member-state that discovered a reportable disease within its borders had a duty to report this to WHO in a timely manner so that action could be taken, if necessary, to minimize the impact and spread of the disease. As such, WHO was designated as *the* technical advisory and conduit for infectious disease control. Due to its legal framework and a desire not to contravene Westphalian principles of non-intervention, the international organization was only able to receive reports from sovereign states. However, examples began to emerge of states delaying reports due to fears of economic repercussions on travel and trade (Cash and Narasimhan 2000). It became clear that there was a bottleneck in the system because if a state chose not to report, there existed no alternative means through which WHO could get hold of the necessary information or act to prevent further spread (Youde 2012: 125). Thus the WHO was powerless to control the international spread of disease in these circumstances.

The reconceptualization of infectious disease as a security threat, as well as other mitigating factors, led to one response in the 1990s – the creation of the Global Public Health Intelligence Network (GPHIN) by the Public Health Agency of Canada (PHAC) in 1997. Its mandate was to track outbreaks that may not have been reported to WHO and to offer effective real time surveillance. Furthermore, when the World Health Assembly (WHA) passed resolution 54.9 (2001), it gave WHO the authority *to collaborate with all potential partners in the area of epidemic alert and response.* This gave WHO the mandate to do what it was already doing unofficially: using non-state and digital disease surveillance systems, such as GPHIN as well as other information coming from states, sub-national agencies, non-governmental organizations, individuals, news reports, or internet sources as it saw fit (Mack 2006: 373). The inclusion of non-state actors like GPHIN multiplied the sources of surveillance information available to WHO and was the catalyst for the creation of the Global Outbreak Alert and Response Network (GOARN) as a repository for epidemic intelligence coming from the range of newly approved sources and a control centre to manage the ensuing response. This was created in the department of Global Alert and Response at WHO to provide a 'network of networks' (Heymann et al. 2001: 348) of WHO collaborating centres working in disease surveillance, verification, and response so as to have a team of experts ready for action, should such a public health event of concern, i.e. a security threat occur.

For Fidler (2004), this incentive for states to report alters the context in which states exercise sovereignty in connection with infectious diseases. Until WHA Resolution 54: 9, and the subsequent revisions to IHR (2005), WHO would not have been unable to use information gleaned from GPHIN (or any other non-official sources) in their global surveillance activities as the information had not been provided legitimately by a member state. Those who heralded the post-Westphalian shift in global health started to suggest that systems like GPHIN and GOARN would 'create a pincer that squeezes the state's sovereign decision whether to report an outbreak or not and forces them to cooperate with WHO' (Fidler 2003: 20). In so doing, fears arose over a shift in the balance of power from the sovereign state to WHO in the realm of disease control. Conversely, this chapter will argue that, in fact, what has occurred is a *resurgence* of the role of the state in global disease surveillance and the gradual retreat of WHO.

This chapter will analyze the role that WHO has played in global disease surveillance to date. It examines this through three key stages of its development: the use of GPHIN as part of the surveillance infrastructure; the shifting responsibilities of GOARN; and finally the waning of both these initiatives, and by extension the prominence of WHO, in disease surveillance and control. This chapter contends that whilst GPHIN and GOARN provide important repositories for disease information and the potential for rapid response in an outbreak, they are no longer as effective as they have been. States have begun to use GPHIN and similar such systems directly, bypassing the role of WHO in this relationship. Additionally, the revisions to the IHR (2005) require individual states to reach a certain capacity for surveillance and response, to do so, states must increasingly manage outbreak responses without WHO. As a consequence, I argue, GPHIN and GOARN have increasingly become the victims of their own success (Kamradt-Scott 2010: 808).

Global Public Health Intelligence Network (GPHIN)

As WHO and several of its member-states began to frame the spread of infectious disease as a security concern, they similarly began to appreciate the necessity of accurate and timely surveillance to have knowledge of any potential threat. They sought approaches to the detection of infectious diseases that were faster than the traditional paper-based route of confirmation of clinical cases from official state sources (Weir and Mykhalovskiy 2010: 80). To this end, WHO started to look outside the established infrastructure of sovereign reporting mechanisms and engaged with an initiative, GPHIN, which was emanating out of Public Health Agency of Canada (PHAC).

GPHIN is a disease early-warning system that seeks to alert its subscribers to a wide range of information about potential outbreaks as close to real-time as possible (Mykhalovskiy and Weir 2006). It does this through a semi-automated software programme which scans a range of news articles (primarily sourced from Factiva and Al Bawaba), and other online sources, including other digital disease surveillance systems like ProMED-Mail, and social media sites, for articles offering information pertaining to unusual disease events based on established search queries. Taking cue from the concept of an 'all risk approach' (Fidler and Gostin 2006: 86) to global health from WHO's IHR (2005) revisions (including human, animal, and plant health), these search queries are related to six key areas for news of an outbreak: infectious diseases; biologics; chemical; environmental; radioactive; and natural disasters (Mykhalovskiy and Weir 2006: 43).

The initial concept was developed in response to overlapping concerns about dramatic increases in the scale and pace of international travel, the limitations of established WHO coordinated surveillance systems, and the official notification of outbreaks being outpaced by the widespread emergence of online global health news (Weir and Mykhalovskiy 2006).

During the plague outbreak in Surat, India, in 1994, Canadian public health officials realized they had more information than either the Indian government or WHO thanks to the combined efforts of CNN and an individual Indian doctor who communicated epidemiological data with them daily. Canadian health officials saw the potential of such informal data-sharing and began developing a more formal model (GPHIN interview; Weir and Mykhalovskiy 2006). This marked an important shift in surveillance, as policymakers began to understand that surveillance needed a more global approach that could bypass the state entirely. This could prevent an outbreak from spreading beyond international borders and reduce the harm inflicted on trade and travel security – even if a state continued to withhold information. Thus, Public Health Agency of Canada saw that the improvement of surveillance technology would allow harvesting and centrally collating considerable information from a range of actors with considerable public health benefit. States could not prevent the collection of this information, as it was open sourced or volunteered by individuals. It was up to GPHIN to assess and verify these data. The value of this network was demonstrated when the system identified an outbreak in Guangdong province, China, as early as November 2002 – more than 2 months before the WHO publicly published details on cases of the new respiratory illness later defined as Severe Acute Respiratory Syndrome (SARS) (Wilson and Brownstein 2009: 829).

Although automation is a key component to the timeliness of the system, GPHIN also employs trained analysts to provide essential linguistic, interpretive and analytical expertise. Out of the estimated 2,000–3,000 sources processed daily, up to one-third of these are then scrutinized in relation to their relevance to previous events; wider trends in infectious disease movements; and the political or socio-economic impact of regions where pathogens may have been found. It is then decided which news stories are worthy of being shared with the wider GPHIN community (Mykhalovskiy and Weir 2006: 43). These analysts add a human element to understand the context in which the outbreak is occurring, and thus limit the risk of releasing false information (Interview B 2012).

What was significant about the emergence of GPHIN in the global disease surveillance landscape at that time was its unprecedented relationship with WHO. In 1999, WHO and Public Health Agency of Canada agreed that GPHIN would provide WHO with all its disease monitoring data and that WHO would use this information as the foundation for wider disease control efforts. This was solidified by both the changes to the WHO's surveillance capacity in WHA 54.9 and the revisions to the IHR (2005). Although GPHIN was not expressly named in either of these documents, their work is documented as one of the most important sources of informal information related to outbreaks on WHO's website – the only intelligence source listed by name. WHO was at the centre of this disease surveillance information system, offering leadership in verifying information and response to assist in cases of an outbreak, of vital significance as the state in question would not necessarily be privy to the information of the outbreak any earlier than the team in Geneva. This positioned WHO in a new role beyond that of a technical advisor – a real-time epidemic intelligence coordinator (Kamradt-Scott 2010: 809). GPHIN's technology is precisely what gave WHO this initial power.

GPHIN reports are shared with WHO and other GPHIN subscribers; and recently the system has moved from a subscriber only service to becoming an open source (no fee) surveillance provider (Davies 2012: 98).

Even before the outbreak of SARS, the Canadian government was already a leader in using web-based surveillance technologies to forecast potential socio-economic collapse (Aginam 2004: 208; Wilson and Brownstein 2009). GPHIN drew on this legacy, and brought together the resources of the Centre for Emergency Preparedness and Response, Public Health Agency of Canada, and the wider Canadian government. The Canadian government sees its creation of GPHIN as part of a wider contribution to international society (CAHS 2009: 6). Several public health professionals at WHO and other governments view GPHIN as a more reliable source of non-state disease surveillance simply because it is coordinated by a government (Interview D 2012).

Several researchers have concluded that GPHIN and its relationship with WHO constitute a transformation in the social organization of knowledge of international infectious disease outbreaks (Davies 2012; Heymann and Rodier 1998; Weir and Mykhalovskiy 2010). First, GPHIN has sped up epidemiological analysis at the international and national level. Using the news as the basis for detecting outbreaks has replaced lengthy and time-consuming paper-based surveillance operations. This has been a centrepiece in WHO's change in institutional thinking from 2000s onwards towards *early detection* and *rapid response*. Second, prior to GPHIN, sovereign nations controlled what information they shared with WHO (Weir and Mykhalovskiy 2006). GPHIN was the first of its kind in this new wave of non-state disease surveillance, and it challenged the sovereign decision making right of nation states to decide when to report an outbreak to the international community. With the information it has collected readily available to WHO, GPHIN could be seen to apply pressure on a government to report an outbreak sooner than it might otherwise intend (Fidler 2004: 65).

Global Outbreak Alert and Response Network (GOARN)

The Global Outbreak Alert and Response Network (GOARN) is a network established by WHO in 1997 and formalized in 2000. The network interlinks in real time a large number of existing institutions which together possess the requisite data, expertise, and skills needed to keep the international community ready to respond to an unexpected disease event (Heymann et al. 2001: 348). Its raison d'être was to take disease reports from a range of sources (including GPHIN) and connect the dots in an attempt to verify and respond to outbreaks from the earliest possible moment (Grein et al. 2000: 97; Sturtevant et al. 2007: 119; Youde 2012: 200). It consists of over 250 institutions including other UN agencies, ministries of health, academic institutes, WHO regional offices, and reference laboratories – all ready to form field response teams, if the host state consents, to coordinate the diagnosis of virus strains and send rapid response teams for disease containment and treatment (Heymann et al. 2001: 350; Davies 2011: 432). WHO envisioned that GPHIN would provide raw epidemic intelligence data that GOARN would then use to verify with the country in question and initiate an effective containment response.

Whilst originally established as a body to coordinate both surveillance and response at the WHO level, GOARN's focus has shifted towards response. Epidemic intelligence is still being carried out by the GOARN team, but it constitutes a small part of their work (Interview B 2012). GOARN's surveillance activities rely upon two main sources of information. The first is its Event Management System (EMS) for outbreak surveillance. This system links WHO HQ, regional offices, and member-states as a forum for information sharing. Here any rumours of unconfirmed clusters or confirmed outbreaks are shared so all members-states who have signed up to the IHR (2005) can see the relevant news or latest actions taken by WHO as a consequence. As GOARN is managed by WHO, the GOARN Secretariat is also privy to EMS information. The second area is digital disease surveillance systems such as Healthmap, ProMED Mail, and GPHIN, which have become increasingly competitive in this area in recent years.

Once GOARN receives outbreak related information, it is then analysed to assess the probable timeframe, mortality, risk of economic loss, potential for affected vulnerable populations, capacity of health systems in the region, and implications for international health security (Interview A 2012). Thus, like GPHIN, there is a considerable need for human analysts to be able to consider these factors. Whilst GOARN has proven an effective coordination tool for sharing information and initiating a response to a suspected event, the priority for GOARN when they hear rumour of a new potential outbreak is to get effective epidemiological analysis and laboratory confirmation: this is where the network comes into its own. The network is able to contact the host state's Ministry of Health and assess the capacity of the public health infrastructure and offer the support of the wider GOARN network of epidemiologists, disease specialists and laboratories if necessary so as to understand the extent of the outbreak as soon as possible (Interview A 2012).

Critics allege that diseases surveillance and response systems focus on diseases that only pose a risk to Western states (Ingram 2009: 2085; Leach 2010: 3 72; Weir and Mykhalovskiy 2006: 259). However, GOARN was set up to focus on viral haemorrhagic fevers in Africa, and subsequently expanded its remit to include the rest of the world (Sondorp et al. 2011: 32). Thus, what the critics miss here is that the landscape of disease surveillance and response is a dynamic process that had to start at some point, but which is becoming increasingly global. Moreover, GOARN has begun to veer into advocacy as much as it does technical coordination and assistance. In recent years, the mechanism has served to highlight a burden of diseases in which the frequency or extent may not have been fully established. GOARN has supported bringing to the attention of policymakers and the global community those preventable diseases that risk being overlooked due to political or budgetary constraints. For example, GOARN brought attention to Nodding Disease in Uganda, which subsequently led to the first high-level WHO meeting on the disease in 2012 (WHO 2012a).

As posited by Davies (2010: 41), WHO is plagued by three key problems: politics, funding, and position – and GOARN, as a WHO institution, is no exception to these. Politics have stymied GOARN as it has tried to improve its systems to ensure global health security. In 2009, it attempted to coordinate a meeting of all disease surveillance providers to establish a more cohesive system among them in order to promote greater health security. Whilst initially there was political will to improve such interconnectedness, the outbreak of H1N1 that same week halted these efforts. As a result, the motivation to improve surveillance was sidelined, and the potential for a stronger coordinated infrastructure led by WHO through GOARN has not materialized. Funding has also caused problems for GOARN. Due to the financial crisis and changes to the departmental objectives in which GOARN sits (Health Security and Environment), the initiative has seen its budget greatly reduced. Although this has not affected the quality of the partners who action the response, it has put considerable pressure on the limited coordinating team in Geneva (Interview B 2012). Finally concerning position, the institutions that form GOARN have over time developed their own relationships with each other independently of

WHO, thus reducing GOARN's central coordinating position in this structure. There have been several instances of member states contacting these institutions bilaterally for support with their disease control without involving the WHO multilaterally. Whilst this is not true for all member states, and there is still considerable coordination carried out by the GOARN team, the role of GOARN may continue to be sidelined accordingly as relationships are further established. Additionally, when examining the outbreak of H5N1 between 2004 and 2008, the response effort has included a much wider range of actors, including the Food and Agriculture Organization (FAO), the Organization for Animal Health (OIE), and the World Bank. Moreover, with the creation of a whole new UN body to manage influenza outbreaks, the United Nations System Influenza Coordination (UNSIC), GOARN and WHO saw their role in disease management further reduced (Kamradt-Scott 2010: 809).

Gone?

WHO was originally designated as *the* technical agency for global health. In terms of disease control, it has certainly played a critical role in the development of a global framework for surveillance and response. While there is no single institution or agency that has the capacity to tackle all infectious disease events (Roth 2006: 100), WHO has been able to achieve the goals of its *early detection and rapid response* approach by bringing partners together through GPHIN and GOARN (Interview A 2012). When technology for disease surveillance was in its infancy, GPHIN was a leader in the field and formed a historically novel reporting relationship with WHO. However, the mechanisms of GPHIN and GOARN as leaders in international surveillance are fading with the resurgence of the state at centre-field. The influx of non-state actors in disease surveillance and member-state's increasing capacity in disease outbreak response have made member-states less reliant on GPHIN and GOARN, and, more broadly, WHO.

First, there are now a variety of surveillance providers building on the initial concept developed by GPHIN. These other data sources include digital disease surveillance providers such as ProMED Mail, CIDRAP, and HealthMap, which member-states have favoured using as part of wider post-2008 budgetary austerity WHO programmes (Interview E 2013). There is also a net of NGOs, civil society groups, and contacts working the field (Interview C 2012). As a key informant discussed 'It is not the digitalization of disease surveillance per se which has changed the manner in which the international community learns of outbreaks, but the revolution in information technology means that anyone can communicate with colleagues, officials and the WHO instantaneously' (Interview G 2013). Instead of relying on the tracing of media sources alone as pioneered by GPHIN, the opportunity has also arisen to share information directly with contacts globally who then might be able to implement a response quicker than if they went through the GPHIN and GOARN procedures. This has in turn led to a reduced role for these institutions and, more generally WHO.

Second, Article 5 of the IHR (2005) requires member states to 'develop, strengthen and maintain ... the capacity to detect, assess, notify and report events in accordance with the regulations'. Whilst a considerable number of member states have asked for an extension past the 2012 deadline for implementation, a significant percentage of states have begun the process and have improved their capacity for surveillance and response considerably (WHO 2012b) and thus are less reliant on the support of GOARN. In many respects, the consequence of the revised IHR (2005) has been to – in the long term – reduce the demand for GOARN (IHR 2005; Kamradt-Scottt 2010). This was compounded with the third event, the Global Financial Crisis. The global economic recession has led to an underfunding of WHO and restrictions on how the organization uses its funds, which in turn further marginalizes GOARN (WHO 2011).

These three factors combined have meant that states have begun to manage outbreaks independently without WHO's involvement other than their notifying obligations to the organization. Additionally, states have entered into bilateral agreements with GOARN member institutions directly, such as with the United States' Centers for Disease Control and Prevention, France's Institut Pasteur, or Germany's Robert Koch Institute (Interview B 2012). Although all data collected independently or bilaterally under the IHR (2005) is shared with WHO, this can be seen as a mere function of their duties as responsible states (Davies and Youde 2013: 137) rather than as a precursor for a response.

Notwithstanding international pressure to upgrade surveillance and response capabilities in all countries (under IHR 2005 revisions), vast disparities remain evident in both domains and the globe remains unprepared for an all-too-plausible global health scenario (Ingram in Pain and Smith 2008: 81). Developing states are starting to include wider digital disease surveillance systems as a low-cost option for improved disease control, but expanding internet access in many areas is prohibitively expensive (Sturtevant et al. 2007: 117). Conversely, Western states have started to use non-state sources in order to guarantee their own health security when the WHO system is unable to provide the requisite information in a timely manner. Thus we need to consider how such state behaviour informs states' intelligence-gathering exercises and not just analyse the role and impact of GOARN or GPHIN in a vacuum (Davies 2012: 107).

Even WHO itself admits that states still do not rely on their system for outbreak alert and response because it lacks credibility as an authoritative source (WHO 2011: 13). Member-states agreed to and ratified the revisions to the IHR (2005); therefore, they should be confident that all states will comply with them and report diseases occurring amongst their populations to WHO. If this system were functioning as intended, then individual states would be able to rely solely on WHO and therefore would not need to carry out their own epidemic intelligence within their Ministries of Health or have their own individual subscriptions to other digital disease surveillance systems. The question that arises is, are states expanding the surveillance playing field because they do not trust that the WHO system is working effectively, they do not trust other states' reporting standards, or even their own capacity to respond to an outbreak? In each case, the point remains that (Western) member states have moved away from relying on WHO in disease surveillance, and as such WHO does not enjoy the prominent role in surveillance that it did a decade ago.

As Lee highlights, WHO has continually been caught between the utopian health of all peoples and the *realpolitik* of having to engage with reluctant state actors (Lee 2009: 9). GPHIN and GOARN are no exception to this tension. The rise of such global initiatives does not necessarily indicate that states are failing to detect and respond to outbreaks themselves; rather, they show that traditional governance mechanisms cannot always satisfy the novel and all-encompassing global dimensions of emerging diseases alone. In fact, governments have supported the use of networking (GOARN) and technology (GPHIN) as a way of improving their own surveillance infrastructure at the national and international levels (Khoubesserian in Cooper and Kirton 2009: 288). For example, states like the United Kingdom and France have begun issuing press releases specifically so that they will be picked up by GPHIN and other disease surveillance mechanisms, although rarely is this reported by those analysing such systems. This creates a different perspective on the global disease surveillance landscape, if in fact, the signals are coming from the state in the first instance (Davies 2012: 107). This reality problematizes the notion that states are still seeking to hide information from the global community, and inflates the intelligence capacities of digitalized systems (such as GPHIN), when the actor's progress on surveillance that we need to observe are the governments making this information available (Davies and Youde 2013: 146). Again, this points to the continuing reality that states themselves remain the vital player in disease surveillance, even with the increase of non-state digital disease surveillance providers.

Globalization is often linked with weakening the power of the state. In global health, this includes introducing non-state actors to the landscape and encouraging new links between the private and public sectors in the search for creative ideas and greater efficiency in governance (Long 2011: 65). However, disparities exist between academic interpretations of non-state actors and their real appearance in the global health setting. For example, some commentators have suggested that as an example of globalization, the creation of GOARN as a network of various actors has created a system of global emergency vigilance which changes public health reasoning to constitute WHO as a super sovereign power (Weir and Mykhalovskiy 2010: 141). However, in actual fact, whilst the activities of GPHIN and GOARN discussed are symptomatic of such creative ideas for greater efficiency, this does not mean that WHO is necessarily the central tenet of such a governance landscape. With the introduction of a plethora of other actors and increased information technology competing for the work of GOARN and GPHIN, WHO's central status has been weakened. What's more, the role of the state has not been challenged to the extent that is sometimes suggested. It can be said that the changes in the governance structure and legal framework (IHR 2005) reflect the global health governance regime beyond a state-centric model (Youde 2012: 126). Whilst this may be true of the collection of data, this does not mean that the response and sovereign decision-making activity in relation to the information collected has been undermined.

Conclusion

Without a doubt, the role of GPHIN in widening the parameters of global disease surveillance was paramount. It was the foresight of a few key individuals at PHAC who understood the potential of harnessing news information from the internet for public health purposes. This then altered how WHO received information about disease outbreaks to include the media and other non-state sources. The consolidation of GOARN in 2000 to form a networked community of epidemiologists, laboratories and potential rapid response teams to instigate an immediate response mechanism in the case of an outbreak further changed the landscape disease control and WHO's role within it. It brought in a range of partners in a new governance setting in order to provide the best possible service to its member states, and meanwhile enhance global health security.

Although the response to SARS (2002/3) by GOARN and WHO as a whole has been widely commended, it has been described by others as the start of the demise of WHO as the leading institution in disease surveillance and response (Kamradt-Scott 2010: 810). However, this waning of its role in global disease control ought to be understood as a result of its own achievement in this field. Whether intentionally or not, WHO – through its championing of PHAC's GPHIN initiative and the creation of GOARN – initiated a trend in widening the sphere of global disease surveillance. Changes to the IHR (2005) to improve national capacity for disease surveillance and response, as well as the fostering of relationships between different member states and GOARN institutions, mean that states have to become better at managing their own outbreaks and supporting each other bilaterally. With WHO in a less central position we can see that individual states will need to dominate the agenda on the future of global disease surveillance. Summed up, 'states remain the master-builders, but the new management structure is increasingly a device built by many hands pulling many levers' (Simons and Oudraat in Zacher and Keefe 2008: 138). The many hands include the range of actors providing epidemic intelligence and response assistance, yet the state still maintains control of what to do with the information it receives and how to play their sovereign reporting duties accordingly. Of course, not all states can be classed as equals in dominating the global disease surveillance agenda, as a considerable 'surveillance gap' (Fidler 2006: 197) still remains between Western and developing states. Perhaps this is where WHO, and by extension GPHIN and GOARN, can still play a crucial role: in supporting developing states to reach the IHR (2005) required capacity for surveillance and response, providing resources for them to respond to an outbreak, as well as realizing a potential future for greater advocacy in raising the agenda of neglected and chronic disease.

Bibliography

Bashford, A. (ed.). 2006. *Medicine at the Border: Disease, Globalization and Security 1850 to the Present*. New York: Palgrave Macmillan.

Brownstein, J., Freifeld, C., Reis, B., and Mandl, K. 2009. Surveillance Sans Frontieres: Internet-Based Emerging Infectious Disease Intelligence and the HealthMap project, *PLoS Medicine*, 5(7): e 151.

Canadian Academy of Health Sciences (CAHS). 2009. *Canada's Strategic Role in Global Health*, Global Health Symposium Meeting Summary, 21st September 2009. Available at: http://www.cahs-acss.ca/wp-content/uploads/2011/09/CAHS_Global_Health.summary.pdf [accessed 29 July 2013].

Cash, R.A. and Narasimhan, V. 2000. Impediments to global surveillance of infectious diseases: Consequences of open reporting in a global economy, *Bulletin of the World Health Organization*,78(11): 1358–67.

Cooper, A. and Kirton, J. 2009. *Innovation in Global Health Governance: Critical Cases*. Farnham: Ashgate.

Davies, S.E. 2010. *Global Politics of Health*, Cambridge: Polity Books.

Davies, S.E. 2011. The duty to report disease outbreaks, of interest or value? Lessons from H5N1, *Contemporary Politics*, 17(4): 429–45.

Davies, S.E. 2012. Nowhere to hide: Informal disease surveillance networks tracing state behaviour, *Global Change, Peace, and Security*, 24(1): 95–107.

Davies, S.E. and Youde, J. 2013, *The IHR (2005), Disease Surveillance, and the Individual in Global Health Politics*, International Journal of Human Rights, 17(1): 133–51.

Fidler, D.P. 2003. Global Challenges to Public Health: SARS, Political Pathology and the First Post-Westphalian Pathogen, *Journal of Law, Medicine and Ethics*, 31: 485.

Fidler D.P. 2004. *SARS, Governance and the Globalization of Disease*. New York: Palgrave Macmillan.

Fidler, D.P. 2006. 'Biosecurity: Friend of Foe for Public Health Governance?', Bashford, A. (ed.) 2006. *Medicine at the Border*. New York: Palgrave Macmillan.

Fidler, D.P. and Gostin, L.O. 2006 The New International Health Regulations: An historic Development for International Law and Public Health, *Journal of Medicine, Law and Ethics*, 34(1): 85–94.

Grein, T., Kamara, K., Rodier, G., et al. 2000. Rumours of Disease in the global village: outbreak verification, *Emerging Infectious Diseases*, 6(2): 97–102.

Heymann, D. and Rodier, G. 1998. Global Surveillance of communicable disease, *Emerging Infectious Diseases*, 4(3): 362–5.

Heymann, D. and Rodier, G. 2004. Global Surveillance, National Surveillance and SARS, *Emerging Infectious Diseases*, 10(2): 173–5.

Heymann, D., Rodier, G., and the WHO Operational Support Team to the Global Outbreak Alert and Response Network. 2001. Hot spots in a wired world: WHO surveillance of emerging and re-emerging infectious diseases, *Lancet Infectious Diseases*,1(5): 345–53.

Ingram, A. 2009. The Geopolitics of Disease, *Geography Compass*, 3(6): 2084–97.

Interview A, 2012, WHO Geneva.

Interview B, 2012, WHO Geneva.

Interview C, 2012, WHO Geneva.

Interview D, 2012, London.

Interview E, 2013, Health Protection Agency, London.

Interview F, 2013, Ministry of Health, Laos.

Interview G, 2013, London.

Kamradt-Scott, A. 2010. The evolving WHO: Implications for global health security, *Global Public Health*, 6: 8.

Leach, M., Scoones, I., and Stirling, A. 2010. Governing Epidemics in an age of Complexity: Narratives, Politics and pathways to sustainability, *Global Environmental Change*, 20(3): 369–77.

Lee, K. 2009. *The World Health Organization*. London: Routledge.

Long, W. 2011. *Pandemic and Peace: Public Health Cooperation in Zones of Conflict*. Washington: USIP Press.

Mack, E. 2006. The World Health Organization's new International Health Regulations; incursions on state sovereignty and ill-fated response to global health issues, *Chicago Journal of International Law*, 7(1): 365–77.

Mykhalovskiy, E. and Weir, L. 2006. The Global Public Health Intelligence Network and Early Warning Outbreak Detection, A Canadian contribution to global public health, *Canadian Journal of Public Health*, 97(1): 42–4.

Pain, R. and Smith, S. 2008. *Fear: Critical Geopolitics and Everyday Life*. Aldershot: Ashgate .

Rodier, G. 2007. New Rules on international public health security, *Bulletin of the World Health Organization*, 85(6): 428–30.

Roth, C. 2006. Epidemic and Pandemic Alert and Response, *Refugee Survey Quarterly*, 25(4): 100–103.

Sondorp, E., Ansell, C., Hartley Stevens, R., and Denton, E. 2011. *Independent Evaluation of The Global Outbreak Alert and Response Network*, Geneva: World Health Organization.

Sturtevant, J., Anema, A., and Brownstein, J. 2007. The new International Health Regulations: considerations for global public health surveillance, *Disaster Medicine and Public Health Preparedness*, 1(2): 117–21.

Weir, L. and Mykhalovskiy, E. 2010. *Global Public Health Vigilance: Creating a World on Alert*. London: Routledge

Wilson, K. and Brownstein, B. 2009. Early Detection of Disease Outbreaks using the Internet, *Canadian Medical Association Journal*, 180(8).

World Health Organization 2001. *World Health Assembly Resolution 54.9 Global Health Security – Epidemic Alert and Response*. Available at: http://apps.who.int/gb/archive/pdf_files/WHA54/ea549.pdf [accessed 26 June 2012].

World Health Organization. 2005. *International Health Regulations*. Geneva: World Health Organization.

World Health Organization. 2011. *Implementation of the International Health Regulations (2005): Report of the Review Committee on the Functioning of the International Health Regulations (2005) in Relation to Pandemic (H1N1) 2009*, 64th World Health Assembly, 5th May 2011 Provisional Agenda item 13: 2. Available at: http://apps.who.int/gb/ebwha/pdf_files/WHA64/A64_10-en.pdf [accessed 1st August 2013].

World Health Organization. 2012a. *Regional Office for Africa, Nodding Syndrome Meeting, researchers agree on case definition and establish research agenda*, 1 August 2012. Available at: http://www.afro.who.int/en/uganda/press-materials/item/4826-nodding-syndrome-meeting-researchers-agree-on-case-definition-and-establish-research-agenda.html [accessed 12 December 2012]

World Health Organization. 2012b. *Implementation of the International Health Regulations (2005)*, Executive Board: 132 Session Provisional Agenda Item 8.1, 21 December 2012.

World Health Organization. 2013. *Global Alert and Response: Epidemic Intelligence, Systematic Event Detection*, available at: http://www.who.int/csr/alertresponse/epidemicintelligence/en/ [accessed 9 August 2013].

Youde, J. 2012. *Global Health Governance*. Cambridge: Polity Books.

Zacher, M. and Keefe, T. 2008. *The Politics of Global Health Governance: United by Contagion*. New York: Palgrave Macmillan.

Chapter 8

Insights into Surveillance from the Influenza Virus and Benefit Sharing Controversy

Frank L. Smith III

Introduction

Pandemic influenza is one of the most prominent threats on the agenda for the World Health Organization (WHO), prompted in large part by fears about H5N1 influenza. A critical component of the WHO response to potential pandemics is its Global Influenza Surveillance Network (GISN), which helps monitor flu viruses and manufacture vaccines. In 2006, however, Indonesia stopped sharing its samples of H5N1 with GISN until wealthy countries and industry started sharing drugs and other benefits in return. The resulting controversy over virus and benefit sharing challenged longstanding norms about disease surveillance, and years of contentious negotiations were required to reach agreement on a new Pandemic Influenza Preparedness Framework in 2011.

What caused this controversy, and why is it important? Indonesia's defection from GISN is difficult to dismiss or discount, since it experienced the most virulent strain of H5N1 and the highest proportion of human cases. This chapter therefore provides a historical overview of the initial response to H5N1 in Indonesia. The controversy over virus and benefit sharing is shown to be a distributional conflict, triggered by inequitable access to drugs and unfavorable reporting. This pitted the national interests of Indonesia and other poor countries against wealthy countries like the United States and the commercial interests of industry. This chapter charts how countries like Indonesia appeal global cooperation that they observe as failing in benefit to their particular situation.

Given this distributional conflict of interests, what lessons can be learned about disease surveillance, global norms, and international law? First, Indonesia's defection from GISN suggests that surveillance behaves like a luxury good, whereas the conventional wisdom simply assumes that it is a global public good. Both may be true, but this controversy illustrates how the information provided by surveillance is of little benefit without the material resources—including but not limited to drugs—that are necessary for public health action. Indonesia appeared to place a higher priority on drugs than surveillance, while wealthy states demanded surveillance because they already had the other resources required to put this relative luxury to use.

Second, the controversy demonstrates that even well-established norms are subject to challenge and change (see Chapter 2). The norm of unconditionally sharing virus samples stood more or less uncontested for more than 50 years, until Indonesia defected from GISN. The interests that motivated this defection were also inconsistent with the altruistic motives that Martha Finnemore and Kathryn Sikkink (1998) associate with the "norm life cycle," and the normative dynamics at play imply that "tipping points" and "cascades" may be poor analogies as well. Moreover, the appropriateness of some norms is no guarantee that the benefits of surveillance outweigh the opportunity costs, particularly if the information it provides is a luxury for some states.

The last lesson addressed in this chapter is that legal arguments are both ubiquitous and epiphenomenal. Not only was international law equivocal and inconclusive throughout this controversy; the new framework that supposedly resolves virus and benefit sharing is too weak to change the status quo. Consequently, international law is unlikely to compensate for the inequitable distribution of material resources across the income divide between wealthy and poor states. These are discomforting lessons to learn, since they all suggest that distributional conflicts will continue to fester long after this particular controversy fades from view.

Conflicts of Interest Over Avian Influenza

The virus at the heart of this controversy is H5N1, which is a highly pathogenic avian influenza. It first crossed the species barrier in 1997, when H5N1 infected at least 18 people and killed six in Hong Kong. Although no new human cases were discovered for the next several years, the virus continued to circulate and spread through the bird population. It re-emerged in people in 2003 and, since then, human cases have been reported every year. As of August 2013, more than 600 laboratory-confirmed cases of H5N1 have occurred, with the highest proportion of cases concentrated in Indonesia (WHO 2013). By that same time, more than 350 people had died from this disease worldwide, which equates to a frightfully high case fatality ratio of nearly 60 percent. It is even worse in Indonesia, where this ratio exceeds 80 percent. Fortunately, however, bird flu remains rare in humans, and there is little or no evidence of sustained person-to-person transmission to date.[1]

Shortly after human cases of H5N1 re-emerged in 2003, WHO started reporting surveillance information and collecting samples of the virus through GISN. This network was officially established in 1952 and, as one of several types of surveillance, GISN represents a series of exchange relationships between states,

---

1   Human transmission has probably caused one or more clusters of cases (especially among members of the same family), but it is rare and not sustained. See Ungchusak et al. (2005).

WHO, and industry. As shown in Figure 8.1, states collect samples of the "wild-type" flu viruses that circulate in their populations. Traditionally, they share some of these samples with WHO Collaborating Centres, which are large laboratories like the Centers for Disease Control and Prevention (CDC) in the United States. WHO Collaborating Centres use these virus samples to analyze the evolution of influenza, identify which strains to vaccinate against, and formulate "seed strains" of the viruses to target with vaccines. The seed strains are then distributed to industry, which use them to manufacture vaccines.

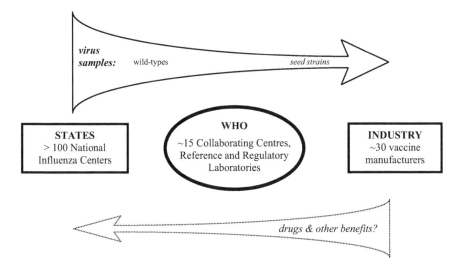

Figure 8.1   **Exchange relationships within the Global Influenza Surveillance Network (recently renamed the Global Influenza Surveillance and Response System)**[2]

By coordinating all of this activity, GISN has long served as an important focal point in the fight against seasonal influenza, and it started to do the same with H5N1. However, as this virus spread and fear of a pandemic grew, GISN became a flashpoint for conflict over the distribution of vaccines and other benefits that are derived from shared virus samples. This distributional conflict came to a head in 2006, when Indonesia stopped sharing its samples of H5N1 with GISN. But tension had been building since 2005, when the first human cases of avian influenza appeared in Indonesia. The origins of this controversy can therefore be traced back to Indonesia's discontent over the difficulty of acquiring drugs and unfavorable reporting about H5N1.

---

2   WHO (2009; 2012; 2012).

The Indonesian government had difficulty acquiring the antiviral drug oseltamivir (sold by Roche under the brand name Tamiflu®) to treat its initial cases of H5N1. At the time, oseltamivir was in short supply and wealthy countries had bought what little was available to stockpile as a precautionary measure—even though, unlike Indonesia, they were yet to suffer any human cases of bird flu. This inequitable distribution of drugs angered the Indonesian Minister of Health, Dr. Siti Fadilah Supari, and helped set the stage for future conflict (Supari 2008).

As H5N1 became increasingly prevalent in Indonesia, Supari increasingly found fault with reporting by WHO. In particular, several members of an Indonesian family died from H5N1 in May 2006, after which WHO reported that these cases might represent the first known instance of human-to-human transmission (Bird 2006; McNeil 2006). Supari protested against this suggestion, which she interpreted as a slanderous and inaccurate accusation that could damage Indonesia's economy—let alone her reputation as Minister of Health (Supari 2008: 16–18).

This dispute over unfavorable reporting helped turn virus samples into a point of political contention.[3] Supari assumed that genetic testing would vindicate her protest, even though WHO never said that human-to-human transmission was due to genetic mutation. Since genetic data about the virus samples shared through GISN were restricted to a few databases with limited access, Supari started to support transparency and oppose GISN (Enserink 2006: 1224). For example, she disclosed some sequence data about the Indonesian strain of H5N1 on a public access database in August 2006, and she was initially praised in the Western media for sharing this information (*The Economist* 2006).

Praise soon turned to condemnation, however, when Supari decided to stop sharing virus samples with GISN in December 2006. The timing is unclear, but either immediately before or shortly after making this decision, Supari discovered that an Australian company was developing a vaccine based on the Indonesian strain of H5N1—using seed stock provided by a WHO Collaborating Centre (the U.S. CDC), without express permission from the Indonesian government.[4] This discovery dovetailed with discontent over Indonesia's inability to acquire oseltamivir and the dispute over unfavorable reporting, so it provided Supari with further justification to withhold virus samples. Thereafter, Indonesia's defection from GISN was described as a protest against the lack of benefit sharing by the pharmaceutical industry in wealthy states:

> Disease affected countries, which are usually developing countries, provide information and share biological specimens/virus with the WHO system; then pharmaceutical industries of developed countries obtain free access to this

---

3   For a related explanation but distinct lessons, see Elbe (2010).

4   Accounts vary on when Supari decided to withhold virus samples, as well as on when she learned about the Australian company's H5N1 vaccine. See Sedyaningsih et al. (2008: 486) and Supari (2008: 35–7).

information and specimens, produce and patent the products (diagnostics, vaccines, therapeutics or other technologies), and sell them back to the developing countries at unaffordable prices. (Sedyaningsih et al. 2008: 486)

Indonesia therefore refused to share its virus samples through GISN unless and until WHO distributed the benefits derived from these samples in a more equitable manner. Indonesia acquired several allies in this call for reform, but it was not the only state that withheld H5N1—China also hoarded avian and human samples—and the resulting controversy served other interests as well (Branswell 2007). By focusing attention on WHO, for example, this controversy served Indonesia's interest in limiting or distracting from unfavorable reporting about the prevalence of H5N1 inside its territory. Likewise, Iran supported Indonesia, in part because it was an opportunity to oppose the United States (regardless of the merits of reform) (Supari 2008: 66, 75). Other members of the Non-Aligned Movement also voiced their support for reforming GISN, as did several likeminded countries like Brazil.

Other interests aside, Indonesia and its allies wanted to reform GISN in order to gain greater access to vaccines and other technology. Consequently, they sought to create an explicit and enforceable link between the virus samples that states share through GISN and the benefits derived from these samples—particularly the vaccines manufactured by the pharmaceutical industry. One way to recognize this chain of rights and obligations is through a Standard Material Transfer Agreement (SMTA), which is a type of legal contract. SMTAs usually function as contracts in private law, which differs from public international law between states. Nevertheless, Indonesia and its allies wanted these contracts to govern exchanges between state laboratories, an international organization (WHO), and third parties (i.e. industry).

Opposing these reforms were wealthy states like the United States, along with the pharmaceutical industry. They preferred the *status quo ante*, when virus sharing was unconditional and uncoupled from benefit sharing. According to the U.S. Secretary of Health and Human Services, "the issues of the availability of vaccines and the sharing of samples are both legitimate ones, and we must deal with them both, but we should not link. World health should not be the subject of barter" (Leavitt 2008). As a result, the United States initially opposed using SMTAs. It later sought to restrict these contracts to the transfer of wild-type viruses from states to WHO, excluding transfers from WHO to industry, so as to neither obligate industry to share benefits nor impinge on the intellectual property rights for technology derived from shared virus samples. Opponents argued that such a contract would only amount to a meaningless "shipping document," but, like the United States, pharmaceutical manufactures also favored a narrowly defined SMTA (Shashikant 2009).[5]

---

5   On the International Federation of Pharmaceutical Manufacturers and Associations, see Mara (2009).

Negotiations over these controversial reforms were "a long and arduous process" (Chan 2009). WHO officials started negotiating with Supari before her decision to defect from GISN in 2006, but countless meetings and years of debate seemed to produce little progress, even after Supari was replaced as Indonesia's Minister of Health in 2009. However, in April 2011, a WHO working group finally agreed on a new Pandemic Influenza Preparedness Framework, which was adopted the following month by the World Health Assembly.

This framework changed the name of GISN to the Global Influenza Surveillance and Response System (GISRS), and it addressed virus and benefit sharing through SMTAs. As I will soon discuss, however, marginal changes in process and naming should not be confused with substantive changes in outcome. So what lessons can be learned from this framework and the distributional conflict that preceded it? In particular, what insight does the controversy over virus and benefit sharing provide into disease surveillance?

Surveillance as a Luxury Good

Perhaps the most important lesson from this controversy is that disease surveillance appeared to behave like a luxury good.[6] This conclusion complicates the conventional wisdom, which tends to sideline analysis of the costs and benefits of surveillance by simply championing it as a global public good.[7] In theory, pure public goods are non-rival (their use by one person does not prevent others from using them) and non-excludable (their benefits cannot be denied, even to people who do not pay). Everyone therefore has an incentive to free ride rather than pay, so providing public goods is a collective action problem.

Once they are provided, however, benefiting from public goods is not typically treated as a problem. But if disease surveillance through GISN was a pure public good, with non-rival consumption and non-excludable benefits, then how could benefit sharing become controversial in the first place? The notion of non-excludable benefits is particularly puzzling in the context of this controversy. How could distributional conflict even arise, if the benefits provided by surveillance were readily accessible to everyone?

As these questions suggest, this controversy confounds the simplistic assertion that surveillance is a global public good. Although the information provided by surveillance is non-exclusive when widely reported, it is only beneficial when acted upon to treat the sick and control the spread of infection. A pharmaceutical response involving vaccines and antiviral drugs is only one of several options; other public health actions include sanitation and hygiene, as well as quarantine, social distancing, and using personal protective equipment. Yet whatever form they take,

---

6   Similar conclusions are reached—using different evidence—by Calain (2007).

7   See Fidler (2004: 66). For a more sophisticated but still contestable assessment, see Woodward and Smith (2003: 14).

medical treatment and infection control always require material resources—drugs, medical manpower, and the like—beyond mere information.

Additional resources are therefore necessary in order to benefit from surveillance. If these resources are more important for public health action than the information provided by surveillance, then surveillance will probably behave like a luxury good. A luxury good is defined by how demand for the material or service in question responds to differences in income: surveillance is a luxury if demand for this information increases disproportionately to an increase in income (i.e. if wealthier states want it far more than the poor). Luxury goods and public goods are not mutually exclusive categories, however, because public goods vary along a variety of different dimensions, including their income elasticity of demand, as well as their utility and expense.[8]

Qualitative evidence from the controversy considered here suggests that surveillance behaved like a luxury good, at least when demand for it is compared with the concurrent demand for drugs. First, both wealthy and poor countries wanted drugs. Wealthy countries stockpiled oseltamivir, for example, just as Indonesia tried to acquire the same drug to treat H5N1, even though it is a poor country. This suggests that demand for drugs was relatively income inelastic, meaning that it was insensitive to large differences in national wealth.

In contrast, poor countries were not as infatuated with surveillance as wealthy countries like the United States, which could afford to put such a luxury to use. The difference in demand across the income divide is illustrated by Indonesia's defection from GISN and the fact that American officials condemned this decision as a threat to global health (see Leavitt 2007). Although GISN represents only one type of surveillance, it is instructive because the virus samples involved are needed to create vaccines (unlike other types of surveillance, where the link to medical treatment and infection control is more tenuous). To a greater degree than demand for vaccines and other drugs, even demand for this type of surveillance was sensitive to differences in national income; perhaps disproportionately so, like a luxury good. Moreover, Indonesia's decision to withhold its virus samples until it received more substantive benefits—placing surveillance at risk—was also consistent with the fact that information alone is of little benefit.

Second, demand for drugs was very sensitive to the prevalence of disease. International demand for oseltamivir shot up in the face of a potential H5N1 pandemic, as did demand for vaccines once they were available. This relationship is a defining feature of economic epidemiology, which argues that "the price elasticity of demand is lower the more demand responds to disease occurrence" (Geoffard and Philipson 1997: 222). In other words, if the prevalence of disease drives up the demand for drugs, as seen here, then demand for those drugs stands

---

8 If surveillance is expensive, then it might resemble the public good of national defense (see Smith 2010: 7). Likewise, if demand for surveillance is income elastic, then it might resemble the public good of a lighthouse that is in disproportionate demand by people wealthy enough to travel by boat.

to be relatively insensitive to how much they cost. This relationship provides further support for the previous point; namely, that demand for drugs was income inelastic. It is also consistent with the claim that Supari was initially frustrated by the insufficient supply of oseltamivir as much as by its high price. "Even when the fund[ing] was in hand," Supari (2008: 5) argued, Indonesia still could not satisfy its demand, "because the medicine had been purchased by developed countries for stockpiling"—this is not to say that price was not a factor as well.

Yet the demand for surveillance appeared to respond differently than demand for drugs relative to the prevalence of disease. Although global demand for surveillance may have increased with the spread of avian influenza, the incidence of disease complicated if not diminished demand by Indonesia, where H5N1 was most prevalent. At the very least, Indonesia had a disincentive to report the incidence of disease because it might damage travel and trade. This is one reason why noncompliance with the old International Health Regulations (IHR) was routine (Fidler 2004: 35)—and to some extent, the same remains true today. For example, open source evidence suggests that Indonesia may have failed to report several human cases of H5N1 and thereby violated the revised IHR, even after these new regulations entered into force.[9] Supari also sought greater control over the diagnosis of H5N1—at some cost—by transferring this responsibility from the US Naval Medical Research Unit to the Indonesian Ministry of Health. Indonesia is not unique in this regard. Reportedly, Britain and Spain refused to closely monitor the H1N1 pandemic in 2009 and thus violated the revised IHR, which requires that states "communicate to WHO timely, accurate and sufficiently detailed public health information" (Cheng 2009; WHO 2008).

These potential violations of the IHR suggest that states remain sensitive to paying a price in terms of travel and trade when they supply surveillance information. This may affect the level of detail that states demand when collecting information at home, as well as what they eventually report to WHO. Granted, states also pay a price for drugs, but they appear more willing to do so—even when it imposes painful tradeoffs on poor countries. In Indonesia, it was "with much difficulty," according to Supari (2008: 5), that "the government tried to split its budget to buy the medicine." Nevertheless, Indonesia was more willing to buy medicine than pay the potential price of publicly reporting surveillance information. Once again, this suggests that poor countries see drugs as a necessity relative to surveillance, which they see as a luxury.

In sum, even if disease surveillance is a global public good, it may also behave like a luxury good, since information requires additional resources in order to be

---

9   See Roos (2008; 2009). Alternatively, Indonesia may have reported these cases to WHO and this information was kept confidential, in which case Indonesia may not have violated the IHR (depending on the timing). But confidential information is exclusive—contrary to the definition of a public good. This would also challenge the claim that WHO provides "human security" (rather than national security), since confidentiality would mean reserving information for states rather than reporting it directly to the public.

of much benefit or use. This creates several problems. For instance, poor countries are less inclined to pay for luxury goods by definition. Even if they do, these states cannot benefit from the information that surveillance provides without the other resources required for medical treatment and infection control. Although surveillance can assist in the efficient distribution of limited resources, its benefits should be weighed against the opportunity costs of collecting this information and not merely assumed to be self-evident, as simplistic rhetoric about public goods might otherwise suggest. Stated differently,

> the reason for collecting, analyzing and disseminating information on a disease is to control that disease. Collection and analysis should not be allowed to consume resources if action does not follow. Appropriate action, therefore, becomes the ultimate response goal and the final assessment of the earlier steps of a surveillance system. (Foege et al. 1976: 30)

Dynamic and Dubious Norms

What does demand for luxury goods imply for the normative dynamics surrounding surveillance? This controversy considered here demonstrates that the norms inherent to international regimes like GISN are not immune to challenge. Paradoxically, challenge is integral to the notion of a "norm life cycle." According to Finnemore and Sikkink (1998: 897–8), this cycle only begins when "norm entrepreneurs" challenge established practices and promote alternative ideas, motivated by factors like altruism and empathy.

Perhaps Supari was a norm entrepreneur, but her decisions were motivated in part by the national interests at stake in a distributional conflict over material resources. These resources appeared more useful than the relative luxury of surveillance and, as a result, Supari violated the norm of unconditionally sharing viruses: a practice that had seemingly been internalized and taken for granted for more than 50 years. Given delayed reporting of H5N1, Indonesia's compliance with the revised IHR is also questionable and thus might challenge yet another set of surveillance norms. Even if these challenges and violations were exceptional, they are difficult to disregard because Indonesia was such a hotspot for H5N1.[10]

Therefore, the extent to which supposedly global norms govern state behavior remains an open question, long after they seem to have cascaded past some tipping point into common practice. Here "tipping points" and "cascades" are poor analogies, since they are associated with irreversible transitions, followed by rapidly accelerating rates of change. This controversy challenges both the

---

10   Nor can Indonesia be dismissed as a rogue state. Not only was "internationalism" a sanctioned philosophy (*pancasila*) when it won independence; Indonesia was also a driving force behind the founding of the Association of Southeast Asian Nations, and it remains so to this day.

irreversibility and acceleration of norms relating to virus sharing and surveillance, as well as benefit sharing. A more apt analogy might be critical junctures, punctuated by either reversals or ratchet effects. Critical junctures—or "turning points"—provide a more accurate account than the tipping points proposed by Finnemore and Sikkink, particularly when the cusp of change is defined by an exogenous shock (e.g. the outbreak of H5N1, SARS, or another disease), rather than the internal momentum of a given norm.

Norms relating to surveillance will survive this particular controversy and, in time, some might become increasingly habitual, obligatory, or appropriate (see Chapter 2). But appropriate is not the same as "good," especially if surveillance behaves like a luxury good. For example, consider fashion. People are often obligated to wear fashionable ties or high heel shoes, yet it is hard to argue that these norms are beneficial or good, even when they are appropriate or habitual.[11] Disease surveillance is certainly more substantive than many fashions and fads, but the information that it provides is still no substitute for action—even if states are socialized to see some norms about monitoring and reporting as appropriate.

Limits of International Law

In 2011, after years of negotiations, WHO Member States finally agreed upon a new Pandemic Influenza Preparedness Framework. Among other provisions, this framework attempts to resolve the controversy over virus and benefit sharing by infusing these processes with legal contracts. Therefore, is international law likely to solve the problems associated with surveillance as a luxury good? Being so new, any conclusions about this framework are inherently speculative, but the controversy that preceded it illustrates how international law rarely governs state behavior. Although international law figured prominently in this controversy, it was equivocal and inconclusive. For its part, the new framework also appears far too weak to compensate for the inequitable distribution of benefits derived from surveillance.

Looking back, almost every question in this controversy was subject to legal debate. For example, did Indonesia violate international treaty law by defecting from GISN? On one hand, "Indonesia's actions would not violate the IHR," since these regulations can be interpreted as only requiring states to communicate public health information—not share biological material like virus samples (Fidler 2007). On the other hand, the United States argued that withholding virus samples was "inconsistent with the spirit" of this treaty, and the Director General of WHO reportedly "said that countries that do not share avian influenza virus would fail

---

11   Early arguments about the logic of appropriateness did not conflate "appropriate" with "good," since it was recognized that historical inefficiency can produce suboptimal outcomes. See March and Olsen (1998). Unfortunately, subsequent scholarship tends to confuse appropriateness with desirability or even morality.

the IHR" (Leavitt 2007: 1763). There is a legal basis for this interpretation as well, since the IHR obligates states to facilitate the transport of biological substances and support WHO response activities—both of which could apply to GISN (WHO 2005: Articles 46, 13).

Customary law is even less conclusive than treaty law. It can be argued that defection from GISN did not violate customary international law because states never shared virus samples out of a sense of legal obligation (also known as *opinio juris*) (Fidler 2007). The definition of this motivation is contested, however, and customary international law also rests on established state practice—like the decades of practice that Indonesia departed from by withholding virus samples (Goldsmith and Posner 1999).

Similar debates played out over linking virus and benefit sharing through Standard Material Transfer Agreements. For example, Indonesia and its allies argued that these contracts were required by the Convention on Biological Diversity (Sedyaningsih et al. 2008: 487). SMTAs also appear consistent with other treaties, including the International Seed Treaty. But U.S. officials and others argued that the Convention on Biological Diversity was inapplicable, since H5N1 was initially seen as a threat to biological diversity and an invasive pathogen rather than an indigenous organism (Fidler 2009: 91). The precedent provided by the International Seed Treaty can be debated as well, since its SMTA contains features that are "totally unique and without precedent in international law" (Chiarolla 2008: 7).

International law was therefore equivocal and inconclusive, almost without exception. Indeed, states engaged in "norm shopping," whereby they chose from among numerous norms and legal arguments, selecting only those that supported their self-interests.[12] Given international anarchy, there was no overarching authority to arbitrate between these different legal norms, let alone to force states to adopt or comply with any particular interpretation of law. WHO was certainly too weak to do so; as an international organization, it moderated this dispute but lacked the power and autonomy needed to resolve the underlying conflicts of interest between states.

Looking forward, the Pandemic Influenza Preparedness Framework will probably do little to ameliorate these conflicts or change the balance of power between states, industry, and WHO. Though celebrated as a "landmark agreement," this celebration is more about ending years of controversial negotiations rather than the content of the framework itself (WHO 2011). In short, the framework recognizes rights and obligations regarding virus and benefit sharing through two SMTAs: one for transfers between states and the WHO Global Influenza Surveillance and Response System, and another contract for transfers from GISRS to outside parties like industry. It also requires industrial partners to pay half the

---

12 Norm shopping is so common that is taken for granted, even though this term—analogous to "forum shopping"—is rarely used. For a similar usage and definition, see Posner (1997: 367).

operating cost of GISRS, which currently amounts to an annual contribution of about 30 million U.S. dollars (WHO 2011: 18). Finally, the framework acknowledges that virus and benefit sharing are equally important, and it affirms norms like transparency, as well as equitable access to drugs and other technology.

Nevertheless, even advocates for a legalistic approach to global health governance acknowledge that this framework is relatively weak and does little to alter the status quo (Fidler and Gostin 2011: 200–201; Enserink 2011: 525).[13] In particular, it imposes few if any legally binding obligations on state governments. States "should" share viruses according to the framework, just as they "should urge" industry to distribute drugs and other benefits in an equitable manner, but states are not actually required to do anything.

While the framework does not bind states, it does impose obligations on other actors (namely, WHO and industry). For industry, these obligations are incurred—but not enforced—through SMTAs that make only the vaguest references to dispute resolution, let alone to potential penalties for breaches of contract, and the obligations are minor. For example, contributing a few million dollars towards the operating cost of GISRS represents little more than a rounding error for multinational corporations that earn billions of dollars a year from drugs and diagnostics. For better or worse, this is probably one reason why industry endorsed this weak framework. It also enjoys industry support because the framework supports intellectual property rights. States are encouraged to respect these rights but discouraged from claiming them on virus samples, whereas industry is free to pursue intellectual property rights for the technology it derives from shared samples. Industrial partners are obligated to share some drugs or other benefits, but only during a potential influenza pandemic (which occurs, on average, only once every few decades). Moreover, they can share these benefits in any number of small ways, most of which are consistent with industry donations prior to this framework.

So little that triggered this controversy or transpired during it would violate the framework that supposedly resolves virus and benefit sharing. This suggests that international law will likely remain indeterminate if not irrelevant. Perhaps Indonesia and others that favored reform won a procedural victory through this framework by adding a legal patina to the status quo. This might affect the *process* of disease surveillance through the use of SMTAs, sample tracking, and the like by GISRS. However, important *outcomes* appear unlikely to change, particularly those that relate to medical treatment and infection control. As a result, the public good of surveillance will probably remain of little consolation to poor countries that lack the basic goods and services needed to take full advantage of it.

---

13   For a useful critique, see Kamradt-Scott and Lee (2011).

A Discomforting Reality

Any single case study has its limitations. Nevertheless, the lessons to be learned from this controversy do not bode well for international law or the other norms that surround surveillance. Legal arguments were epiphenomenal, states broke established international norms, and surveillance itself appeared to behave like a luxury good. Disease surveillance is informally defined as "information for action," but, as shown here, conflict over the resources required for public health action can threaten both the supply and relevance of information itself.

This fundamental problem is acknowledged—but not solved—by the weak attempt to link virus and benefit sharing through the Pandemic Influenza Preparedness Framework. This framework will fail to change the status quo because international law rarely if ever does and, more important, wealthy states like the United States oppose substantive change. Wealthy states can afford to use surveillance information, which is why they probably want it more than the poor, yet even the wealthy do not want it at any cost, and certainly not at the cost of their drug supply. Information is desirable but, for rich and poor alike, it stands to be secondary to demand for the material resources that states need to act in response to a potential pandemic. As a result, distributional conflicts over drugs and other resources will likely persist as defining features during the response to transnational outbreaks of infectious disease.

Acknowledgements

The author would like to thank participants of the July 2011 "Politics of Disease Surveillance Workshop," especially Sara Davies and Jeremy Youde, as well as Charles Belle, Simon Bronitt, Ian Hall, and Andrew O'Neil.

References

Branswell, H. 2007. With Indonesian Bird Flu Standoff in the Spotlight, China Still Hoards Viruses. *The Canadian Press* [Online, 15 April] available at: http://www.canada.com/topics/news/world/story.html?id=e45b07ae-111e-4d3b-b24a-aee0349ea59f&k=40072 [Accessed: 3 December 2012].

Calain, P. 2007. From the Field Side of the Binoculars: A Different View on Global Public Health Surveillance. *Health Policy and Planning*, 22 (1), 13–20.

Chan, M. 2009. Opening remarks at the Director-General's Consultation with Member States on Pandemic Influenza Preparedness. *Intellectual Property Watch* [Online, 19 October] available at: http://www.ip-watch.org/weblog/wp-content/uploads/2009/10/chan-flu-speech-oct-09.pdf [Accessed: 7 November 2011].

Cheng, M. 2009. UK's Attempts to Stop Swine Flu Called Flawed. *Guardian* [Online, 21 May] available at: http://www.guardian.co.uk/world/feed article/8519949 [Accessed: 4 December 2012].

Chiarolla, C. 2008. Plant Patenting, Benefit Sharing and the Law Applicable to the Food and Agriculture Organization Standard Material Transfer Agreement. *The Journal of World Intellectual Property*, 11 (1), 1–28.

CNN. 2006. Bird Flu Scare: Human Spread? *CNN* [Online, 24 May] available at: http://articles.cnn.com/2006–05–24/health/indonesia.birdflu_1_human-to-human-transmission-bird-flu-h5n1?_s=PM:HEALTH [Accessed: 6 November 2011].

Elbe, S. 2010. Haggling over Viruses: The Downside Risks of Securitizing Infectious Disease. *Health Policy and Planning*, 25 (6), 476–85.

Enserink, M. 2006. As H5N1 Keeps Spreading, A Call to Release More Data. *Science* 311 (5765), 1224.

____. 2011. "Breakthrough" Deal on Flu Strains Has Modest Provisions. *Science*, 332 (6029), 525.

Fidler, D.P. 2004. *SARS, Governance and the Globalization of Disease*. New York: Palgrave Macmillan.

____. 2007. Indonesia's Decision to Withhold Virus Samples from the World Health Organization: Implications for International Law. *American Society of International Law Insights*, 11 (4), 1–6.

____. 2008. Influenza Virus Samples, International Law, and Global Health Diplomacy. *Emerging Infectious Diseases*, 14 (1), 88–94.

Fidler, D.P. and Gostin, L.O. 2011. The WHO Pandemic Influenza Preparedness Framework: A Milestone in Global Governance for Health. *JAMA*, 306 (2), 200–201.

Finnemore, M. and Sikkink, K. 1998. International Norm Dynamics and Political Change. *International Organization*, 52 (4), 887–917.

Foege, W.H., Hogan, R.C. and Newton, L.H. 1976. Surveillance Projects for Selected Diseases. *International Journal of Epidemiology*, 5 (1), 29–37.

Geoffard, P. and Philipson, T. 1997. Disease Eradication: Private versus Public Vaccination. *The American Economic Review*, 87 (1), 222–30.

Goldsmith, J.L. and Posner, E.A. 1999. A Theory of Customary International Law. *The University of Chicago Law Review*, 66 (4), 1113–77.

Kamradt-Scott, A. and Lee, K. 2011. The 2011 Pandemic Influenza Preparedness Framework: Global Health Secured or a Missed Opportunity? *Political Studies*, 59 (4), 831–47.

Leavitt, M. 2007. *Statement on the World Health Assembly Resolution on Pandemic Influenza Preparedness: Sharing of Influenza Viruses and Access to Vaccines and Other Benefits*. [Online: US Department of Health and Human Services] available at: http://www.hhs.gov/news/press/2007pres/05/pr20070523a.html [Accessed: 7 November 2011].

Leavitt, M. 2008. Secretary Mike Leavitt's Blog. [Online: US Department of Health and Human Services] available at: http://archive.hhs.gov/secretarys blog/my_weblog/pandemic_planning/index.html [Accessed: 6 November 2011].

Mara, K. 2009. Officials Working Informally Towards May Consensus on Avian Flu Preparedness. *Intellectual Property Watch* [Online, 8 April] available at: http://www.ip-watch.org/2009/04/08/officials-working-informally-toward-may-consensus-on-avian-influenza-preparedness/ [Accessed: 4 December 2012].

March, J.G. and Olsen, J.P. 1998. The Institutional Dynamics of International Political Orders. *International Organization*, 52 (4), 943–69.

McNeil, D.G. 2006. Bird Flu Case May Be First Double Jump. *New York Times* [Online, 24 May] available at: http://www.nytimes.com/2006/05/24/world/asia/24birdflu.html [Accessed: 2 December 2012].

Posner, R. 1997. Social Norms and the Law: An Economic Approach. *American Economic Review*, 87 (2), 365–9.

Roos, R. 2009. Indonesia Reports 20 H5N1 Cases—19 fatal—since January. *CIDRAP News* [Online, 30 December] available at: http://www.cidrap.umn.edu/cidrap/content/influenza/avianflu/news/dec3009indo.html [Accessed: 4 December 2012].

Sedyaningsih, E.R., Isfandari, S., Soendoro, T. and Supari, S.F. 2008. Towards Mutual Trust, Transparency and Equity in Virus Sharing Mechanism: The Avian Influenza Case of Indonesia. *Annals Academy of Medicine Singapore*, 37 (6), 482–8.

Shashikant, S. 2009. WHO: Key Elements of Virus and Benefit-sharing Framework Still Unresolved. *South –North Development Monitor* [Online, 19 May] available at: http://www.twnside.org.sg/title2/intellectual_property/info.service/2009/twn.ipr.info.090506.htm [Accessed: 3 December 2012].

Smith, F.L. 2010. Look But Don't Touch: Overemphasis on Surveillance in Analysis of Outbreak Response. *Global Health Governance*, 3 (2), 1–15.

Supari, S.F. 2008. *It's Time for the World to Change (in the Spirit of Dignity, Equity, and Transparency): Divine Hand Behind Avian Influenza*. Jakarta: PT Sulaksana Watinsa.

The Canadian Press. 2008. Indonesia Assures It Will Report Bird Flu Cases. *The Canadian Press* [Online, 13 June] available at: http://www.ctvnews.ca/indonesia-assures-it-will-report-bird-flu-cases-1.302253 [Accessed: 28 November 2012].

The Economist. 2006. A Shot of Transparency—Global Health. *The Economist* [Online, 12 August 12] available at: http://www.economist.com/node/7270183 [Accessed: 3 December 2012].

Ungchusak, K., Auewarakul, P, Dowell, S.F., et al. 2005. Probable Person-to-Person Transmission of Avian Influenza A (H5N1). *New England Journal of Medicine*, 352 (4), 333–40.

Woodward, D. and Smith, R.D. 2003. Global Public Goods and Health: Concepts and Issues, in *Global Public Goods for Health: Health Economic and Public Health Perspectives*, edited by R.D. Smith et al. New York: Oxford University Press.

World Health Organization. 2008. *International Health Regulations* (2005). Geneva: WHO Press.

____. 2009. *Influenza Vaccine Manufacturers*. [Online] available at: http://www.
who.int/csr/disease/influenza/Influenza_vaccine_manufacturers2009_05.pdf
[Accessed: November 7 2012].

____. 2011. *Landmark Agreement Improvises Global Preparedness for Influenza
Pandemics*. [Online] available at: http://www.who.int/mediacentre/news/
releases/2011/pandemic_influenza_prep_20110417/en/index.html [Accessed:
7 November 2011].

____. 2011. *Pandemic Influenza Preparedness: Sharing of Influenza Viruses and
Access to Vaccines and Other Benefits*. [Online] available at: http://apps.who.int/
gb/ebwha/pdf_files/WHA60/A60_R28-en.pdf [Accessed: 4 December 2012].

____. 2013. *Cumulative Number of Confirmed Human Cases of Avian Influenza
A(H5N1) Reported to WHO, 2003–2013*. [Online] available at: http://www.
who.int/influenza/human_animal_interface/EN_GIP_20130829CumulativeN
umberH5N1cases.pdf [accessed 3 September 2013].

____. 2012. *Global Influenza Surveillance and Response System (GISRS)*. [Online]
available at: http://www.who.int/influenza/gisrs_laboratory/en/ [Accessed: 7
November 2012].

____. 2012. *WHO Collaborating Centres Global Database*. [Online] available
at: http://apps.who.int/whocc/List.aspx?cc_subject=Influenza& [Accessed: 7
November 2012].

Chapter 9

Biosurveillance as National Policy: The United States' National Strategy for Biosurveillance

Jeremy R. Youde

It may not have come with a grand unveiling during a well-attended press conference from the Rose Garden of the White House, but the National Strategy for Biosurveillance could potentially change how the United States government conceptualizes disease surveillance and the health/security nexus. With its release on 31 July 2012, the National Strategy for Biosurveillance (NSB) began the process of being translated from strategic plan to operational program. The NSB appears to be one of the first times, if not the first time ever, that a national government has adopted a conscious, public strategy that explicitly connects its biosurveillance activities to broader national security strategies. In his introductory letter, Obama explicitly emphasizes that the National Strategy for Biosurveillance builds on the United States' existing security strategies to protect human, animal, and plant health. In this way, the National Strategy for Biosurveillance goes beyond the surveillance requirements mandated by the International Health Regulations to explicitly integrate biosurveillance into a state's larger security and operational apparatuses.

The inauguration of a biosurveillance strategy by a sovereign state raises a host of interesting issues and questions about the relationship between national and international disease surveillance strategies, the intersection of health and security, collaborations with existing surveillance systems, and the financial implications of creating and sustaining such a system. It also forces us to ponder the scope and operation of such a system. Ultimately, the emergence of a national biosurveillance plan forces us to consider whether this is a move that is both appropriate and beneficial. While the United States' program is far too new to allow for definitive conclusions, its creation and initial plans provide an appropriate venue for considering these questions. Further, it connects to larger issues raised by other chapters in this book by examining changes in the modes of biopolitical surveillance and response in the post-IHR (2005) international environment.

This chapter proceeds in three parts. First, it examines the outlines of the National Strategy for Biosurveillance as explained in its July 2012 release report. Second, it considers how the explicit meshing of health and security will work under this system and examines some of the tensions that may arise. Finally, it concludes by discussing the prospects for the National Strategy for Biosurveillance and the likelihood that it will play a significant role in American health policy efforts.

The National Strategy for Biosurveillance

Aside from a short press release from the White House on 31 July 2012, the US government announced the brand new National Strategy for Biosurveillance (NSB) with little fanfare. *Defense Daily*, an online news source focused on defense and aerospace issues, carried a short article about the NSB a week later (Biersecker 2012), and the US Department of Defense's (DoD) Armed Forces Press Service released a statement that highlighted how existing DoD operations would fit with the NSB's planned operations (Pellerin 2012). Otherwise, though, the announcement received little attention from print, broadcast, or online news sources.

In some respects, the National Strategy for Biosurveillance fits in with the minimum core surveillance capacities required by the updated International Health Regulations. Signatories to the IHR pledge to develop and maintain certain key abilities that are necessary for allowing a global all-risks approach to disease surveillance properly operate. These core competencies include:

- national legislation, policy, and financing to authorize such activities;
- coordination among partners and the establishment of a National Focal Point to handle communications with the World Health Organization;
- surveillance capacities;
- response mechanisms;
- preparedness planning;
- risk communication strategies;
- human resources to carry out the required elements; and
- effective laboratory capacities (World Health Organization 2011: 17–19).

Many of the details described in the National Strategy for Biosurveillance resonate with these required core capacities. Where they differ, though, is in their emphases. The IHR's core capacities are technical in nature (however, see Chapter Two); they mandate that states engage in certain actions to uphold their responsibilities. The National Strategy for Biosurveillance, on the other hand, includes normative elements. By locating the importance of biosurveillance within certain other goals and frameworks, the strategy adds a political element that stakes out a very particular place for biosurveillance within the larger schemata of national and international health policies.

In his introductory letter, President Obama does not lay out the details of the NSB itself, but he provides some measure of context for it. He positions the NSB within the realm of national security. "As a nation," he wrote, "we must be prepared for the full range of threats, including a terrorist attack involving a biological agent, the spread of infectious diseases, and food-borne illnesses" (White House 2012: i). He then connects the National Security Strategy, released in 2010, to biosurveillance and the need to obtain timely information on new and emerging health risks. The NSB, Obama argues, builds upon the National Security Strategy to institutionalize biosurveillance efforts. By coordinating among all levels of government, taking advantage of technological advances, and drawing on existing resources, Obama pledges that the NSB will "meet our shared responsibility and deepen the collaboration we need to keep our country safe and secure" (White House 2012: i). At the end of the brief epistle, the American president charges his national security staff to craft an operational plan within 120 days.

At its outset, the National Biosurveillance Strategy establishes three important facets for understanding its place in the larger national apparatus. First, it explicitly connects biosurveillance with national and international security. Indeed, the very definition of biosurveillance used by the strategy comes from 2007's Homeland Security Presidential Directive-21. It defines biosurveillance as:

> The process of active data-gathering with appropriate analysis and interpretation of biosphere data that might relate to disease activity ad threats to human and animal health—whether infectious, toxic, metabolic, or otherwise, and regardless of intentional or natural origin—in order to achieve early warning of health threats, early detection of health events, and overall situational awareness of disease activity. (White House 2007)

While this definition may not be explicitly security-related, it is noteworthy that the 2007 presidential directive initially relates catastrophic health events to terrorist and WMD attacks before addressing the possibility of naturally-occurring disease outbreaks (White House 2007).

The rapid situational awareness and response activities inherent to effect biosurveillance are similar to the efforts necessary to address "a bioterror attack or other weapons of mass destruction (WMD) threat, an emerging infectious disease, pandemic, environmental disaster, or food-borne illness" (White House 2012: 1). It later describes how the enhanced surveillance capacities will apply to "potential human, animal, or plant health impacts resulting from chemical, biological, radiological, and nuclear (CBRN) and environmental incidents, as well as influenza and other public health trends" (White House 2012: 1). The document further links the threat environment in which the United States exists and biosurveillance needs to operate with the September 11th attacks, the Fukashima reactor meltdown, and synthetic biology (White House 2012: 3). This language gives the NSB a very broad conception of health and health surveillance, but it also diverts away from some of the traditional public health conceptualizations of biosurveillance.

Second, the National Biosurveillance Strategy emphasizes how non-revolutionary it is. It is not a new program or change in direction. Rather, it is a strategy to get existing biosurveillance systems to speak to each other. The NSB praises the "strong foundation of capacity arrayed in a tiered architecture of Federal, State, local, tribal, territorial, and private capabilities," but says that the United States needs "increased integration of effort across the Nation" (White House 2012: 1). This is not to say that no new programs will be needed in order to effectively operationalize the NSB, but it does suggest that the basic elements are largely in place and need relatively minor tweaks to be effective in this holistic sense.

Third, and closely related to the previous point, the National Biosurveillance Strategy emphasizes its cost-effectiveness. Relying largely on existing resources at all different levels of government not only encourages officials to buy in to the strategy, but it also means that there will not need to be significant outlays by the federal government. President Obama and his national security staff are cognizant of the need to minimize the fiscal implications of the NSB. In describing the strategy's ability to leverage existing disease surveillance capabilities, it notes that building on such existing foundations is particularly important "in these fiscally challenging times" (White House 2012: 1). Given budget realities in the United States since the start of the global economic recession in 2008, this is likely a prudent move.

The National Biosurveillance Strategy is not itself an operational document; it lays out principles that will need to be operationalized. To facilitate that process, the NSB offers four Guiding Principles, four Core Functions, and four Enablers for Strengthening Biosurveillance.

Guiding Principles

The Guiding Principles focus on finding ways to ensure that the NSB provides value to decisionmakers at all levels while retaining the dynamism necessary to respond to ever-evolving situations. The first principle is "leverage existing capabilities." This means not just drawing on already-existent resources at various levels of government, but also using electronic resources and social media outlets to facilitate communication across a wide variety of constituencies.

The second principle is "embrace an all-of-nation approach." This idea operates on two different levels; it encourages the use of sentinel observation sites throughout the country to generate a comprehensive overview of the country, and it calls attention to the need to pay attention to human, animal, and plant illnesses. It integrates the ideas of One Health into the strategy, compelling decisionmakers to consider how animal, human, and environmental health work together (Davies 2010).

The third principle is "add value for all participants." This principle calls particular attention to the fiscal resource constraints inherent in American government policy since 2008. The government essentially acknowledges that it cannot offer significantly more dollars for biosurveillance efforts, but is placing additional demands on existing resources. As such, it calls on the operational plan to promote efficiencies and help existing surveillance systems do their work even better.

The final principle is "maintain a global health perspective." Focusing solely on the United States is meaningless and ineffective, since health threats can easily travel and cross borders even before they are recognized. This principle recognizes that America's disease surveillance capabilities must necessarily contribute to the larger international ones. It also calls on existing international systems to work with the network of American surveillance systems (White House 2012: 4–5). While it does not identify specific potential collaborators, the list could include GPHIN (see Chapter 5), BioCaster (see Chapter 6), and GOARN (see Chapter 7).

Core Functions

The Core Functions provide a measure of guidance to those who are tasked with operationalizing the National Strategy for Biosurveillance. Establishing an overall goal of "achiev[ing] a well-integrated national biosurveillance enterprise that saves lives by providing essential information for better decisionmaking at all levels" (White House 2012: 5), the NSB's Core Functions are designed to work together in a dynamic function to make the goal a reality.

The first core function is "scan and discern the environment." This means that any biosurveillance efforts must simultaneously operate on multiple levels. They must search for known pathogens, but also be sensitive enough to detect newly-emerging threats. They must look for threats to human, animal, and plant health. Despite the diverse array of environments and situations, the NSB's surveillance efforts must also exhibit the ability to assess the significance of any findings and provide policymakers with enough information to prompt appropriate responses without inducing panic.

The second core function is "identify and integrate essential information." As noted in the previous paragraph, surveillance efforts in and of themselves are inadequate without some means of adequately analyzing any information gleaned through these efforts. The NSB calls for the identification of common elements to national public health emergencies. While acknowledging the uniqueness of any particular outbreak, identifying and relying on a standard set of questions can help speed identification of and notification about an outbreak to the proper authorities. This also calls for drawing on the expertise and resources of a wide variety of experts, including public health officials, law enforcement, and medical personnel.

The third core function is "alert and inform decisionmakers." Such alerts are not one-time events; policymakers must be kept abreast of situations as they continue to evolve and develop over time. The NSB stresses, though, that alerting and informing policymakers does not necessarily mean that the government (at any level) must necessarily take action. By providing accurate information and timely updates, the NSB envisions a scenario where officials can make reasoned, rational decisions at the appropriate moment rather than taking action merely for the sake of doing something.

The final core function is "forecast and advise impacts." This function essentially calls on the government to learn. As biosurveillance systems acquire more and more information, the NSB needs to find ways to use those data to refine decisionmaking procedures and better assess the likelihood of negative outcomes from particular outbreaks. Such measures will allow governments to better prepare for outbreaks, reallocate resources as necessary, and come up with realistic "worst case scenario" plans (along with an understanding of the conditions under which such plans would be appropriate). Doing this requires not only computational models and simulations, but also improved human intelligence and professional development.

Enablers for Strengthening Biosurveillance

The four enablers identified within the National Strategy for Biosurveillance focus more on the infrastructural and logistical requirements needed to make the strategy's goals a reality.

The first enabler is "integrate capabilities." As noted before, the NSB recognizes and acknowledges that there already exists a significant number of disease surveillance resources in the United States. The challenge before the NSB, then, is to get those existing resources to communicate with each other in a meaningful way so as to avoid duplicating resources and to identify where gaps in the system exist. This may mean transcending organizational borders and being creative about getting groups to work together. It also provides a place for social media to augment communication efforts and help keep the public at larger informed about changing situations.

The second enabler is "build capacity." The fact that many resources already exist does not mean that the *right* resources exist for a comprehensive biosurveillance regimen. Additional technical systems may be necessary to provide adequate coverage that can address human, animal, and plant health needs. Aside from developing adequate technical capacity, though, an effective biosurveillance system will require a great deal of human capital that receives ongoing, updated training to keep them abreast of the most current information. The system must be able to translate the data it collects into actionable information that is useful to both medical and non-medical decisionmakers (Moore et al. 2013: 29). Mawudeku et al. (Chapter 5 in this volume) highlight the massive staff load required to establish and maintain GPHIN's disease surveillance system, and the NSB would likely experience similar staffing and personnel training requirements.

The third enabler is "foster innovation." Existing scientific techniques may work well for identifying and responding to outbreaks of already-known pathogens, but they may not have the necessary sensitivity to alert policymakers to new outbreaks or mutations. As such, biosurveillance systems require ongoing improvement, and the NSB recognizes the importance of encouraging innovation and providing ways for new tools and techniques to prove their mettle. While bureaucracies often have a reputation for adhering to existing protocols, the unpredictability inherent in biosurveillance situations necessitates a willingness to experiment and encourage news ways of examining data.

The fourth and final enabler is "strengthen partnerships." The federal government may have ultimate authority in the event of a disease outbreak, but it cannot effectively exercise its authority without building reliable connections with all different levels of government, nongovernmental organizations, academia, and the private sector. The NSB positions the federal government as lacking the resources and expertise to unilaterally act effectively. Working with others, the strategy argues, also increases buy-in from other sectors. Pathogens can quickly cross borders, too, so it is of utmost importance that the NSB effectively liaise with counterparts in other countries and at the World Health Organization. This will improve information gathering and the sharing of best practices.

After laying out the basic underpinnings of the National Strategy for Biosurveillance along with its guiding principles, core functions, and enablers and calling for an implementation plan to operationalize the strategy within 120 days, the document ends by reminding the reader of the connections between biosurveillance and the United States' general posture toward national security. "Protecting the health and safety of the American people through a well-integrated national biosurveillance enterprise," it concludes, "is a *top national security priority*" (White House 2012: 8; emphasis added). While acknowledging that natural causes could give rise to a national health emergency, the strategy repeatedly links the need for the NSB to terrorism and the accidental or deliberate use of CBRN weapons.

While the National Strategy for Biosurveillance is not an operational document, it does lay out the general guidelines under which such a strategy should operate. These guidelines give rise to important questions—not just for the United States, but also for the larger biosurveillance enterprise and the role of states vis-à-vis disease surveillance efforts. This chapter will pay particular attention to three areas of possible concern. First, it will examine the potential implications of the tight connections between national security and biosurveillance outlined in the strategy. Second, it will discuss the possibilities for collaboration between the structures outlined by the strategy and existing biosurveillance tools already in operation. Third, it will look at the implications of national governments creating and implementing their own biosurveillance strategies and whether such moves are overall net gains or losses for health protection and promotion at all levels.

Health, Security, and Biosurveillance

The National Strategy for Biosurveillance repeatedly links its efforts at early detection of disease outbreaks to bioterror attacks. When the document lists the potential sources of a health threat to the United States, it invariably leads off with some form of terrorist attack before referencing the natural emergence and spread of an infectious disease, food-borne illnesses, or plant and animal-based diseases. The fact that the NSB draws its inspiration and operational foundation from the United States' National Security Strategy further reinforces the connection between issues of health and the security of the state.

Drawing a tight connection between national security and biosurveillance raises a number of significant questions about the orientation and operational effectiveness of the National Strategy for Biosurveillance. Concerns about the health/security nexus of the NSB tend to focus on three areas. First, there are worries that the emphasis on national security will concentrate attention on diseases and illnesses that could be weaponized to the exclusion of the vast majority of human, animal, and plant illnesses that cause the majority of mortality and morbidity from infectious illnesses. Second, a focus on national security politicizes health in a way that does not serve most people. The politicization of health may bring greater attention from policymakers, but that attention does not necessarily translate into better support or an augmentation in necessary resources. Third, health organizations may lack the expertise and resources to act as effective security actors. Requiring agencies without expertise or mandate on security-related functions to undertake such activities threatens to weaken both the health and security functions of the National Strategy for Biosurveillance.

Distraction from More Pressing Health Threats

Technically, the NSB embraces an all-risks approach to biosurveillance that does not privilege any particular illness or concern. That said, nearly all of the public discussion of this strategy emphasizes its connection to biological terrorism. The prospect of a bioweapons attack against the United States is truly disturbing, and it is wise to establish protocols to enable timely and vigorous responses if and when such an attack were to occur.

Given the intensity of focus on bioterrorism within the NSB, one may naturally think that bioterrorist attacks are frequent and widespread. Much of the public discussion of bioterrorism emphasizes that the danger from such attacks from the relative low-cost and ease of manufacturing such weapons (Selgelid 2007). The evidence suggests otherwise. Carus (2001) investigated 180 uses of biological agents for terroristic or criminal purposes from the 1970s to the 1990s. Of those 180, he found that 137 were either hoaxes or threats with no evidence of any actual ability to carry out such an attack. In another 10 cases, the perpetrators expressed an *interest* in obtaining biological agents, but did not have any means to actually acquire them (Carus 2001: 8). Kelle's (2007: 224) study of the 12 most plausible cases involving the use of biological agents found that a full 25 percent were merely apocryphal. RAND's Database of Worldwide Terrorist Incidents includes more than 40,000 events between 1968 and 2010. Of these, a mere 13 involved biological agents. Of those 13, 9 came from the anthrax mailings in the United States in 2001. The remaining 4—from Brazil, Kashmir, Pakistan, and Venezuela—caused one death and no other illnesses (RAND National Defense Research Institute 2013). Taken together, this suggests that bioterrorism is either far more costly or far more technically sophisticated than previously imagined.

This is not to deny the importance of preparing for any type of terrorist activity, but it does suggest the value in putting those preparations in an appropriate context.

While the emphasis on bioterrorism within the NSB may appear to be out of line with the actual incidence of such attacks, it is in line with the larger themes in the literature on health security. One of the most prominent themes within health security discussions is the importance of protecting the state against outside, likely bioterrorist, threats (Aldis 2008: 371). Aldis also notes that most discussions of health security explicitly link the idea with a state's foreign policy interests. This raises the specter, he worries, of injecting power politics into humanitarian actions, as it may suggest that states will engage in humanitarian actions to address health crises only if they fear that a given outbreak will threaten their interests in international relations (Aldis 2008: 371–2). While separating pure humanitarian actions out from power politics is highly difficult (Barnett and Weiss 2008), drawing too tight a connection between disease surveillance and humanitarianism threatens to make the NSB look simply like another foreign policy tool.

The NSB's emphases also raise questions about whether it focuses its attentions on the right areas. New pathogens are emerging with greater frequency these days—and not merely as an artifact of increased disease surveillance around the world (Morse et al. 2012: 1957). Despite this fact, though, disease surveillance strategies (including the NSB) still generally privilege acute outbreak events and short-term factors over long-term indicators (Dry 2008: 5). They focus more on containment activities rather than prevention. Indeed, Rushton argues that there has been a gradual decoupling of public health prevention and containment over time—even as there has been an increased reliance on public health infrastructures to maintain disease surveillance systems (2011: 785). These sorts of new outbreak events and their short-term consequences, though, are not necessarily aligned with the threats that people experience in their day-to-day lives to their health. Outbreak events generate a lot of attention and media coverage, but they are not necessarily threats to human health. The NSB, drawing tight connections between disease surveillance and bioterrorism, is potentially poised to pay far more attention to potentially weaponizable diseases, like anthrax, botulism, plague, smallpox, and tularemia (World Health Organization n.d.), than diseases like measles, pertussis, and polio, which have technically been eliminated from the United States but still occasionally appear or are resurgent due to decreases in vaccination rates.

It is also worth highlighting the disease surveillance systems generally pay almost no attention to noncommunicable diseases (NCDs). NCDs are not transmitted from person to person, and they generally play out over a long period of time. The World Health Organization generally classifies NCDs into four different categories: cardiovascular diseases, cancers, chronic respiratory diseases, and diabetes (World Health Organization 2013). While WHO ties the emergence of NCDs to lifestyle factors like poor diet, lack of exercise, tobacco use, and excessive alcohol consumption, scholars have increasingly connected NCDs to larger structural and economic factors that limit individual choice and negate personal autonomy for one's health (Glasgow 2009; 2012). These diseases are becoming increasingly important on a national and international level, as they are responsible for more deaths than infectious diseases in all regions of the world except sub-Saharan Africa—and they are expected to overtake communicable diseases and nutrition-related mortality as the leading cause of death in Africa no later than 2030 (World Health Organization 2013). Previously considered diseases of old age and wealth NCDs are afflicting younger, poorer populations, which could in turn disrupt economic development and governance reforms in a number of developing countries (Bollyky 2012). A recent analysis by the World Economic Forum calculates that NCDs will cost the global economy approximately $30 trillion between 2011 and 2030 and raises questions about possible challenges due to related demographic disruptions (World Economic Forum 2011).

Despite the growing proportion of deaths being caused by NCDs and the increased costs associated with them, disease surveillance systems are almost entirely focused on infectious diseases. As noted above, because of their biases toward acute outbreak events and short-term events, disease surveillance systems are of little use capturing NCDs within this framework. Despite the fact that the vast majority of Americans (and indeed, a majority of all persons around the world) will die from a noncommunicable disease and that such illnesses are far more likely to affect a person on a daily basis than anthrax, H1N1 influenza, West Nile virus, or SARS, the NSB appears ill-equipped to address this most pressing health concern. NCDs are unlikely to be the result of a terrorist attack, and they develop slowly over time, so the factors that would likely set off some sort of alarm within a traditional diseases surveillance system will be glossed over in the case of NCDs. This raises questions about whether the investment in the NSB and its attendant monitoring systems will adequately address the greatest health burden that the nation will face.

The Securitization of Health

The National Strategy for Biosurveillance largely conceptualizes disease surveillance as a security issue—both for the United States and the larger international community. As such, much of the initial operational guidance for implementing the strategy flows through the Department of Defense (Moore et al. 2013). While securitizing health and framing it as a health concern may generate greater attention and more resources, such a move comes with its own baggage. McInnes and Rushton write, "What constitutes a 'health security' issues appears to be determine by something other than a 'clear and present' danger to life" (2013: 116). It is this "something other" that can make securitizing health a difficult element of an effective disease surveillance system.

First, health security means many different things to different audiences. There exists no universally agreed-upon definition of health security. As such, the term itself can generate confusion and mistrust. Aldis notes that developing countries have raised concerns about the term, fearing that it could be used as a cover to justify unwelcome interventions (Aldis 2008: 370). Rushton has three common characteristics of health security definitions: a focus on fast-moving pathogens that pose threats to individuals and states; an emphasis on pathogens that could be weaponized; and a focus on severe disease burdens that could have social, political, economic, or military effects on a state or region (Rushton 2011: 780). Even among these similarities, though, he cautions that the shared language of health security "masks deep divisions in aims, methods, and values" (Rushton 2011: 779). Potentially weaponizable pathogens are but a small subset of infectious diseases, and they are far from the most pressing or common health problems facing the vast majority of people—either in the United States or around the world. Connecting health with its potential for negative effects on the state threatens to privilege a certain subset of diseases and does little to address endemic health concerns that have already depressed economic development or state performance. New diseases can certainly pose a substantial threat, but, as noted above, too much of a focus on the new, novel, and quick can distract attention from the more pressing health concerns. In the end, the ambiguity of how health security is defined can lead to a situation in which health itself is subordinated to how powerful security interests interpret a given health concern.

Second, making health a security issue also transforms security itself. Security becomes medicalized, meaning that it gets interpreted using medical analogies and tying to craft a "prescription" to solve the problem (Conrad 2007: 4). Elbe raises the concern specifically in the context of health and security:

> When the domains of health and security intersect, it does not just shape how particular diseases are governed in the international system; it similarly encourages changes to how security is understood, to how security is provided, and indeed who practices security in contemporary international relations. (Elbe 2011: 848–9)

He describes three interrelated processes that give rise to the medicalization of security: defining insecurity as a medical problem; giving medical professionals a greater role in politics; and attempting to secure populations through medical interventions (Elbe 2010: 23–9). In this way, disease surveillance systems explicitly built on a logic of security transform medical and public health professionals into security officers (an issue that will be described in greater detail below) and shape the sorts of recommended interventions. Medical analogies can be helpful in some instances when it comes to security, but security problems rarely lend themselves to a single "prescription" that can be used to "treat" the problem.

Third, the connections between health and security are far more subtle than the rhetoric of security suggests. This is not to say that there exist no connections between health and security; rather, the connections that do exist are far more indirect and diffuse than the emphasis on securitizing health would suggest. In 2000, the United Nations Security Council held a special session devoted entirely to the threats to national and international health posed by HIV/AIDS. This was the first time in the organization's history that it had ever designated a health concern a security threat, and it brought a great deal of attention and resources. More than a decade out, though, evidence suggests that the consensus generated by this high-level attention appears overstated. As early as 2001, David suggested that designating HIV a security issue was wrongheaded because the UNSC's tools for addressing security threats were wholly inadequate and inappropriate to the challenges that the virus actually presented (David 2001). The linkages are far more complex and varied, but the language of security is too blunt an instrument to allow for appreciating the nuances. The language of security predisposes government officials to take certain kinds of responses, but those responses do not necessarily match up with what is needed on the ground. Indeed, they may raise new tensions (McInnes and Rushton 2010: 225–6). Disease outbreaks may generate scarcities and vulnerabilities, but those disease outbreaks are not necessarily related to security itself (Fischhendler and Katz 2013). An outbreak of West Nile virus or Legionnaires' Disease in the United States could lead to shortages of particular pharmaceutical treatments or interrupt certain government and societal activities, but these are not security concerns per se. By explicitly justifying the need for the NSB on security and bioterrorism grounds, the disease surveillance systems are awkwardly placed to respond to these sorts of challenges.

Finally, the process of securitizing health (or any other issue, for that matter) necessarily removes it from the realm of "normal" politics. When a society transforms something into a security issue or threat, it is implicitly and explicitly stating that the normal political realm is ill-equipped to handle the issue. Calling health a security issue casts the issue "as one of an 'existential threat,' which calls for extraordinary measures beyond the routines and norms of everyday politics" (Williams 2003: 514). Ardau (2004) argues that securitization is an inherently negative process because it prioritizes fast-track decisionmaking in order to respond to the immediacy of the threat and it thrives on creating and sustaining an "Other" that is cast as the enemy or an outsider that cannot be tolerated. Such an environment is wholly inappropriate for addressing health issues. While there may be a need to implement short-term and immediate measures to address a disease outbreak, preventing epidemics and protecting against a bioterrorist attack requires long-term and carefully considered strategies. Because microbes can and do cross borders with remarkable ease, governments must by definition collaborate and cooperate in order to stop the spread of any disease; a biosurveillance strategy that focuses only on the United States to the exclusion of the rest of the world is short-sighted at best. That said, securitization's tendency toward dichotomization encourages policymakers to categorize countries as "good" or "bad," "healthy" or "sick." Such bifurcation could work directly in opposition to the need to build cooperative relationships with a wide variety of countries in an effort to keep Americans health. Furthermore, this dichotomization could trickle down to those who fall ill themselves. If the ill become seen as "the enemy" or "the other," it can discourage them from coming forward to seek treatment, which imperils the greater population.

Resources and Expertise

The National Strategy for Biosurveillance empowers public health officials and structures to take on a great deal of responsibility for monitoring infectious diseases and initiating relevant actions to combat their spread. Making this system work, though, depends crucially on the existence of robust and well-supported structures with trained and skilled personnel. The NSB's emphasis on functioning in a highly cost-effective way raises concerns about whether the underlying infrastructure necessary to make the system work exists. Further, the wide diversity of public health offices and laws across the country lead to potential difficulties integrating systems and making sure that information sharing can occur in a timely and mutually intelligible fashion.

At the national level, much of the United States' biosurveillance efforts flow through the Department of Defense. In 1996, Presidential Decision Directive (PDD) National Science and Technology Council (NSTC-7) explicitly expanded the Department of Defense's mission to include disease surveillance. A decade later, the National Security Strategy specifically linked pandemic disease to national security (Moore et al. 2013: 6–7). Despite this long-standing responsibility, the department's ability to carry out the requirements of the strategy is under question. The Department of Defense operated with no official definition of what constitutes biosurveillance until the Deputy Secretary of Defense released interim guidance for implementing NSB in June 2013 (Moore et al. 2013: 8). Further, while the United States is a signatory to the International Health Regulations and its surveillance requirements, but the government has never explicitly authorized the Department of Defense's global health security work (Moore et al. 2013: 19). As a result, existing biosurveillance efforts are largely geared toward ensuring the medical readiness of American troops, and global health security operations largely lack authoritative oversight, effective coordination, and adequate funding (Moore et al. 2013: 82). This setup raises questions about the relative ease and ability of federal officials to implement NSB's requirements.

Public health is largely a state and local government issue in the United States. Under the Constitution, "public health powers are clearly among those powers reserved for the states. As a result, states have primary authority and responsibility to protect the health of the public" (Velikina et al. 2006: 68). The federal government's role in public health focuses more on setting goals, policies, and standards; providing financing; collecting and sharing information; building public health capacity; and managing services (Velikina et al. 2006: 65). This relatively limited role, though, can lead to some confusion as to which agency has which responsibilities. Within the realm of biosurveillance, the Centers for Disease Control and Prevention acts as the federal government's lead agency (Velikina et al. 2006: 70), but the Department of Homeland Security "has broad responsibilities for situational awareness (of which biosurveillance is one dimension) for terrorism threats and events" (Wagner et al. 2006: 183).

It gets more complicated at the state and local levels. Health codes largely fall under the purview of state and local governments. As such, there is a large degree of variation in health codes and how these subnational governments interpret and implement their biosurveillance roles. They may define reportable conditions in different ways, and the manner in which they report the same infectious disease can vary widely. For example, Connecticut requires physicians to report HIV cases, but Hawaiian law mandates that laboratories make such reports using unique identifiers that do not include the patient's name. This variation could vastly complicate efforts to conduct contact-tracing efforts (Velikina et al. 2006: 69). Not every disease is like HIV or comes with its stigma and politicization, but the variation does point to the challenges in working across jurisdictions.

It is also worth highlighting that the National Strategy for Biosurveillance does not include any mention of making additional funds to support its activities available to the various entities responsible for it. Instead, the document emphasizes the importance of drawing on existing resources to make the program efficient and work within existing budgetary limitations. That is not a bad strategy in and of itself; it makes sense to leverage existing resources to advance a larger policy goal. Further, the NSB is not an operational document, so it is possible that additional monies will come available to help support these programs. What is worrisome about the lack of any mention of funding is that there is no guarantee that the state and local entities that currently conduct disease surveillance activities will be able to maintain their existing services, let alone scale them up as need be. "Biosurveillance funding competes for taxpayer-financed funding with myriad other real and perceived needs," Velikina et al. remind us (2006: 82). This runs the risk of turning the NSB into an unfunded mandate and forcing state and local health departments to make tough decisions as they face increasing demands on their relatively limited (and unlikely to grow) budgets.

Previous national biosurveillance efforts suggest that the information-sharing aspects that must happen in order to facilitate effective decision-making are lacking. In 2004, the National Biosurveillance Integration System (NBIS) was created within the Department of Homeland Security to combine and manage the biosurveillance efforts of a variety of different federal offices. Three years later, when Congress created the National Biosurveillance Integration Center (NBIC) as part of the 9/11 Commission Act as a tool for analyzing biosurveillance systems and sending out alerts as needed, NBIS merged its activities with those of NBIC (Jenkins 2009: 2, 6). NBIC contains four critical elements: acquiring data for analysis from partner agencies and offices; leveraging expertise from across its partnerships; getting strategic and operational guidance from its partners; and developing and maintaining information technology capabilities for data collection and analysis (Jenkins 2009: 6). Despite having partnerships with a wide variety of federal offices and having a firm institutional home within the Department of Homeland Security, NBIC and NBIS have found themselves hamstrung. NBIS was supposed to receive raw disease surveillance data from its partner offices for analysis, but it only received final products with the analysis and interpretation done by other agencies. The raw data that are collected earliest and of the most use to NBIC's analysts were not being provided as late as October 2009, even though it was NBIC's statutory mandate to conduct its analysis on these raw data (Jenkins 2009: 11). This facilitated widespread confusion and uncertainty about what NBIC's mission was and undermined the Center's ability to partner with other agencies. It also made it difficult for the Center to attract and retain skilled personnel. The lines of responsibility for national biosurveillance efforts remain murky, with three different Cabinet agencies having responsibility for different elements. The Department of Health and Human Services has primary responsibility for human illness surveillance, while the Department of Agriculture holds primary responsibility for animal and plant surveillance efforts. The Department of Homeland Security has responsibility for bioterror-related biosurveillance, regardless of whether the outbreaks occur in humans, animals, or plants (Jenkins 2010: 2–3).

The problems experienced by NBIC and NBIS reflect larger quandaries about how best to conduct biosurveillance efforts. Despite the importance attached to biosurveillance, there is no real consensus on how best to conduct it. A systematic review of 29 different biosurveillance systems in 2012 found that there is insufficient evidence to know which system works the best (Kman and Bachmann 2012: 1). Without an understanding of best practices, it is incredibly difficult to assess whether the operational plan for NBS will achieve the ambitious goals laid out for it. This is not merely an American problem, though. Around the world, public health biosurveillance capabilities generally run into problems around information sharing, communication among partners and with relevant agencies, and ensuring adequate and even coverage. As such, many states experience difficulties meeting the minimal core biosurveillance competencies specified by the revised International Health Regulations (Morse et al. 2012: 1962). Many governments experience difficulties in getting various technical systems to speak with each other and providing information that can form a firm foundation for making analytical decisions about responding to disease threats.

While much effort has focused on the technical capabilities necessary to create a useful biosurveillance system, technology is not sufficient. An effective disease surveillance system cannot be overly dependent upon technology; a system is only as strong as its human analysts who can interpret information and work with policymakers to make informed decisions (see Chapters 5 and 6 in this volume for a more detailed discussion of the role of human analysts in disease surveillance). Surveillance systems may have picked up scattered information about a new disease spreading in the New York area in 1999, but they lacked the context and nuance to fully appreciate what might be going on. It took a human to connect disease reports among humans and birds and identify West Nile virus as the culprit. Technology may have assisted, but "the intuition of individual practitioners observing seemingly unrelated phenomena proved to be the catalyst for accurate identification of the disease" (Donahue 2011: 4). That means that well-trained and competent human analysts are of utmost importance for the smooth functioning of an effective national biosurveillance system, but the availability of such personnel is questionable at this time (Jenkins 2010).

Conclusion

The National Strategy for Biosurveillance is a unique document in global health. It puts the United States to be on track with its minimum core surveillance capacities as required by the International Health Regulations, but it goes far beyond that by explicitly connecting biosurveillance to issues of national and international security and bioterrorism. It makes a large commitment to cooperation and collaboration among a diverse set of operating systems, but comes with little funding to ensure the effective functioning of the resulting system. It elevates health's status within the pantheon of federal government officials, but it does so in a way that threatens to undermine its efficacy.

Thinking about the best strategy going forward for the NSB is fraught with some difficulty. Because of its particular mission and its connection to national and international security, much about the operational plans for the National Strategy for Biosurveillance necessarily remains shrouded in secrecy. Revealing too much about how this monitoring takes place, what the sensors are looking for, and how decisions are made about when to alert the public will not be publicly be released, as doing so could undermine its ability to protect against a bioterror attack.

Despite these limitations, three potential improvements come to mind. First, the underlying rationale for the NSB would function better if it were grounded in the language of human security rather than traditional conceptions of national and international security. National and international security rhetoric predisposes particular strategies that emphasize weaponizable diseases and infectious diseases that spread quickly. These are surely important, but they are but a small fraction of the health threats that face most Americans. Further, the evidence accumulated since the 1990s about calling health and disease a security issue suggests that the label is too blunt an instrument to mobilize effective responses. A grounding in human security, with its emphases on the issues facing people in their day-to-day lives and the interrelatedness between health and other societal concerns offers a more holistic understanding and a better platform for mobilizing an appropriate response to health concerns.

Second, despite current budgetary austerity in the United States, the efficacy of the NSB necessitates some sort of commitment of additional financial and human resources. Building and maintaining disease surveillance systems is not cheap, and state and local governments are hardly in a position to shoulder these costs on their own. There may be some opportunities to partner with private and nongovernmental organizations, but the potential sensitivity of the data the NSB collects could make such collaborations difficult to facilitate. In addition to funding, disease surveillance systems need resources to hire, train, and retain skilled analysts who can translate the raw data into actionable information. Again, state and local governments are unlikely to possess the necessary resources on their own.

Third, the NSB needs to be more explicit about its connection with international partners. A national biosurveillance strategy that operates in isolation will both be of limited efficacy and replicate too many existing resources. While the NSB makes overtures toward global cooperation and acknowledges the importance of working with partners, the nature of this cooperation remains underspecified. The NSB may be able to tap into existing global surveillance networks to increase its efficacy. Further, it is of utmost importance that the NSB's findings and reports are shared in some manner with international partners. While care will need to be taken to prevent any particularly sensitive information from getting into the wrong hands, effective global disease surveillance depends crucially on information sharing. What is happening in the United States can have an effect on other countries, and what is happening in other countries can have an effect on the United States. The American government should not overlook the vital importance of these global partnerships, as these collaborations will make all parties safer and healthier.

It remains to be seen whether the United States' National Strategy for Biosurveillance is a harbinger of things to come for other states or an outlier that fails to generate significant benefits. For those who believe in the value of infectious disease surveillance, it is heartening to see a national government apparently take the issue to heart. The framing of the strategy, though, gives some pause as to its ability to live up to the promises it makes.

References

Aldis, W. 2008. Health security as a public health concept: A critical analysis. *Health Policy and Planning*, 23: 369–75.

Ardau, C. 2004. Security and the democratic scene. *Journal of International Relations and Development*, 7: 388–413.

Barnett, M. and Weiss, T.G., eds. 2008. *Humanitarianism in Question: Politics, Power, Ethics*. Ithaca: Cornell University Press.

Biersecker, C. 2012. National Biosurveillance Strategy focuses on information distribution. *Defense Daily* [Online, 6 August]. Available at: http://www. defensedaily.com/publications/dd/National-Biosurveillance-Strategy-Focuses-On-Information-Distribution_18726.html (accessed 23 October 2013).

Bollyky, T.J. 2012. Developing symptoms: Noncommunicable diseases go global. *Foreign Affairs*, 91: 134–44.

Carus, W.S. 2001. *Bioterrorism and Biocrimes: The Illicit Use of Biological Agents since 1900*. Washington, DC: National Defense University.

Centers for Disease Control and Prevention. 2013. West Nile virus disease cases and deaths reported to CDC by year and clinical presentation,

1999–2012. Online. Available at: http://www.cdc.gov/westnile/resources/pdfs/cummulative/99_2012_CasesAndDeathsClinicalPresentationHumanCases.pdf (accessed 18 November 2013).

Conrad, P. 2007. *The Medicalization of Society: On the Transformation of Human Conditions into Treatable Disorders.* Baltimore: The Johns Hopkins Press.

Davies, S.E. 2010. What contribution can international relations make to the evolving global health agenda? *International Affairs*, 86(5): 1167–90.

Donahue, D.A., Jr. 2011. BioWatch and the brown cap. *Journal of Homeland Security and Emergency Management*, 8(1): 1–13.

Dry, S. 2008. *Epidemics for All? Governing Health in a Global Age.* Brighton: STEPS Centre.

Elbe, S. 2010. *Security and Global Health.* Cambridge: Polity.

Elbe, S. 2011. Pandemics on the radar screen: health security, infectious disease, and the medicalization of insecurity. *Political Studies*, 59(4): 848–66.

Fischhendler, I. and Katz, D. 2013. The use of "security" jargon in sustainable development discourse: Evidence from the UN Commission on Sustainable Development. *International Environmental Agreements*, 13: 321–42.

Glasgow, S.M. 2009. What goes up: the genesis and context of health reform in Sweden. *Global Health Governance*, 3(1). Online. Available at: http://ghgj.org/Glasgow_What%20Goes%20Up.pdf (accessed 18 November 2013).

Glasgow, S.M. 2012. The politics of non-communicable disease policy. In *The Ashgate Research Companion to the Globalization of Health*, Schrecker, T. (ed.). Farnham: Ashgate.

Jenkins, W.O. 2009. *Biosurveillance: Developing a Collaboration Strategy Is Essential to Fostering Interagency Data and Resource Sharing.* GAO-10-171. Washington, DC: Government Accountability Office. Available at: http://www.gao.gov/new.items/d10171.pdf (accessed 20 November 2013).

Jenkins, W.O. 2010. *Biosurveillance: Efforts to Develop a National Biosurveillance Capability Need a National Strategy and Designated Leader.* GAO-10-645. Washington, DC: Government Accountability Office. Available at: http://www.gao.gov/assets/310/306362.pdf (accessed 20 November 2013).

Kelle, A. 2007. Securitization of international public health: Implications for global health governance and biological weapons prohibition regime. *Global Governance*, 13(2): 217–35.

Kman, N.E. and Bachmann, D.J. 2012. Biosurveillance: A review and update. *Advances in Preventive Medicine 2012*. doi: 10.1155/2012/301408 (accessed 20 November 2013)

McInnes, C. and Rushton, S. 2010. HIV, AIDS, and security: Where are we now? *International Affairs*, 86(1): 225–45.

McInnes, C. and Rushton, S. 2013. HIV/AIDS and securitization theory. *European Journal of International Relations*, 19(1): 115–38.

Moore, M., Fisher, G., and Stevens, C. 2013. *Toward Integrated DoD Biosurveillance: Assessment and Opportunities.* Santa Monica, CA: RAND Corporation. Available at: http://www.rand.org/content/dam/rand/pubs/research_reports/RR300/RR399/ RAND_RR399.pdf (accessed 11 December 2013).

Morse, S.S., Mazet, J.A.K., Woolhouse, M., et al. 2012. Prediction and prevention of the next pandemic zoonosis. *Lancet*, 380: 1956–65.

Pellerin, C. 2012. DoD has running start on biosurveillance strategy. Armed Forces Press Service (Online, 22 August). Available at: http://www.globalsecurity.org/ security/library/news/2012/08/sec-120822-afps01.htm (accessed 23 October 2013).

RAND National Defense Research Institute. 2013. *Database of Worldwide Terrorism Incidents.* http://smapp.rand.org/rwtid/search_form.php (accessed 18 November 2013).

Rushton, S. 2011. Global health security: Security for whom? Security from what? *Political Studies*, 59(4): 779–96.

Selgelid, M. 2007. A tale of two studies: Ethics, bioterrorism, and the censorship of science. *The Hastings Center Report*, 37(3): 37–41.

Velikina, R., Dato, V., and Wagner, M.M. 2006. Governmental public health. In *Handbook of Biosurveillance*, Wagner, M.M., Moore, A.W., and Aryal, R.M., eds. Burlington, MA: Elsevier Academic Press.

Wagner, M.M., Pavlin, J., Cox, K.L., and Cirino, N.M. 2006. Other organizations that conduct biosurveillance. In *Handbook of Biosurveillance*, Wagner, M.M., Moore, A.W., and Aryal, R.M., eds. Burlington, MA: Elsevier Academic Press.

White House. 2007. *Homeland Security Presidential Directive -21* (Washington, DC: White House). Available at: http://www.fas.org/irp/offdocs/nspd/hspd-21. htm (accessed 25 October 2013).

White House. 2012. *National Strategy for Biosurveillance* (Washington, DC: White House). Available at: http://www.whitehouse.gov/sites/default/files/National_ Strategy_for_Biosurveillance_July_2012.pdf (accessed 23 October 2013).

Williams, M.C. 2003. Words, images, enemies: Securitization and international politics. *International Studies Quarterly*, 47(4): 511–31.

World Economic Forum. 2011. Noncommunicable diseases to cost $47 trillion by 2030, new study released today. (Online, 18 September). Available at: http:// www.weforum.org/news/non-communicable-diseases-cost-47-trillion-2030-new-study-released-today (accessed 18 November 2013).

World Health Organization. N.d. Specific diseases associated with biological weapons. Available at: http://www.who.int/csr/delibepidemics/disease/en/ (accessed 18 November 2013).

World Health Organization. 2011. *IHR Core Capacity Monitoring Framework: Checklist and Indicators for Monitoring Progress in the Development of IHR Core Capacities in Member States.* WHO/HSE/IHR/2010.1.Rev.1. Geneva: World Health Organization. Available at: http://www.who.int/ihr/IHR_Monitoring_ Framework_Checklist_and_Indicators.pdf (accessed 20 November 2013).

World Health Organization. 2013. Noncommunicable diseases. Available at: http:// www.who.int/mediacentre/factsheets/fs355/en/ (accessed 18 November 2013).

Chapter 10

Strengthening National Health Systems' Capacity to Respond to Future Global Pandemics

Jennifer S. Edge and Steven J. Hoffman

Introduction

Effective pandemic governance is more important now than ever, especially given that pandemic risk factors like urbanization, hypermobility, trans-border trade, rapid population growth and changes to the environment and food systems have all increased in tandem with the demands of globalization (Lee and Fidler 2007). These transformative global shifts have fundamentally changed the way pathogens are spread around the world and thus challenged the conventional operations of pandemic surveillance systems (World Health Organization 2007b). The World Health Organization (WHO) estimates that newly emerging infectious disease outbreaks in one country are now only hours away from affecting many others. Pandemics previously spread over years (e.g., bubonic plague in the fourteenth century), months (e.g., cholera epidemics in nineteenth century) or weeks (e.g., Spanish influenza of 1918–1919), but in today's globalized world, Severe Acute Respiratory Syndrome (SARS) took only 17 hours to spread half-way around the world from China to Canada. Future disease outbreaks are expected to take similarly short periods before they affect multiple countries across geographically distinct regions (Hoffman 2010). The 2013 outbreak of H7N9 bird influenza in China – which allegedly spread from infected fowl to humans than the H5N1 strain did in 2003 – is a stark reminder that the threat of a pandemic exists as an imminent threat to human health and international security (Wong 2013). Also of notable concern is the fact that more than 30 unexpected outbreaks of previously unknown pathogens and re-emerging diseases were observed in the past two decades alone (World Health Organization 2007b). Although the great majority of new and re-emerging diseases have not caused pandemics, national health systems that can respond adequately to pandemic threats are fundamental to controlling pandemic-prone local disease outbreaks within a country, throughout a region and around the world.

The consequences of not preparing for pandemic diseases can be catastrophic. For example, the 1918–1920 influenza pandemic caused 50–100 million deaths and infected roughly 500 million people worldwide (Johnson and Mueller 2002;

Taubenberger and Morens 2006). Today, scientists predict an influenza pandemic could affect up to 1.5 billion people worldwide, cause up to 150 million deaths, and leave US$3 trillion in economic damages (Hoffman 2010; Wong 2013). Pandemics can halt all travel to affected areas, cause severe economic hardship, and incite international isolation. Although there have been many calls for government-wide pandemic preparedness plans to be developed, there have been tremendous difficulties in coordinating a collective, integrated response across sectors, including sharing information and capacity across jurisdictional borders (such as equipment, expertise, and funding), streamlining financing for public health, and aligning national action plans to meet the guidelines contained in international agreements (Bechard et al. 2013; Hoffman 2010; Kamradt-Scott 2011).

Experiences with SARS (2003), H5N1 (2005), and H1N1 (2009) reveal how responding to pandemics remains a great challenge even for some of the world's most capable and well-resourced health systems (Del Rio and Hernandez-Avila 2009; Office of the Provincial Health Officer of British Columbia 2010; Salaam-Blyther 2009). For example, after H1N1, it was found that the Canadian federal government's ability to coordinate an effective national response to pandemics was impaired by a lack of health human resources, standardized processes for rapidly setting priorities, and availability of contingency funds (Public Health Agency of Canada 2010). In the United States, national public opinion polls found that a substantial proportion of the public may not have taken the H1N1 vaccine because they did not believe the virus posed a serious health threat. In fact, only 1–3% of those surveyed obtained a prescription for or had purchased antiviral drugs despite the fact that they were thought to be effective in treating potential infections and the risk of H1N1 infection was thought to be high (Salaam-Blyther 2009; Steel-Fisher et al. 2010). In Mexico, delays in reporting and identifying H1N1, combined with the country's uneven public health infrastructure, prevented full information dissemination to all members of the public, particularly those living in rural areas (Ear 2011). Pandemic planning across North America was predicated on the assumption that future outbreaks would originate in birds from another continent (e.g., from Asia). H1N1's North American, non-avian origins caught pandemic response leaders by surprise (United States Department of Health and Human Services 2012). Challenges faced by less resourced countries are naturally even greater.

The local consequences of a pandemic are complex to manage given that unpredictable increases in patient volumes force local healthcare institutions to rely on surge capacity to manage the rise in demand for health services (e.g., rapid re-assignment of beds and conversion of some to intensive care unit spaces, and re-directing sick persons away from primary care to triage facilities) (Elharram et al. 2013). Acute care hospitals in Canada's Province of Ontario, for example, usually function at more than 90% capacity; during an influenza pandemic, they can expect to experience an increase of 25% or more in demand for inpatient and intensive care hospital beds and assisted ventilation services (Zoutman et al. 2010). Any inefficiencies in how patients are assessed and treated within hospital emergency departments represent an even more strenuous burden than usual. Limited surveillance capacity and conflicting views about roles and responsibilities among all healthcare actors and the general public also represent major challenges (Elharram et al. 2013). In sum, demands for healthcare during pandemics can be expected to vastly exceed health systems' capacity, even in the wealthiest jurisdictions (Toner et al. 2006).

Taking the above elements into consideration, in this chapter, we aim to identify three approaches to strengthening health systems' capacity to respond to emerging pandemics and outline key implementation considerations at various levels of governance. We begin by identifying and defining the breadth of challenges associated with pandemics for health systems, and the evidence available to strengthen responses to them.

The problems posed by pandemics are complex, diverse, and multi-dimensional. These include inadequate systems of governance, difficulty sharing information in a timely manner, coordination problems among jurisdictions, competing perspectives across the animal-human health divide, and antimicrobial resistance, well-covered in previous chapters of this book. But policy responses to these problems are further challenged by two complicating developments: 1) a realization that the risk and protective factors for pandemics are changing; and 2) recognition that existing pandemic plans and health system arrangements, programs and strategies are sub-optimal.

Risk and Protective Factors for Pandemics are Changing

The world is experiencing unprecedented levels of change in almost all sectors of society as a result of globalization. The most effective pandemic responses will likely be those that can be customized to address the unique conditions surrounding context-specific cases of pandemic emergence. National and international decision-makers have struggled to link local and global scales of action and transition to a governance paradigm that is inclusive of bottom-up approaches (Wilbanks and Kates 1999). The global response to H1N1, for example, has been criticized for following a one-size-fits-all approach (Day 2013). Current pandemic prevention and management efforts do not all account for the dynamism and diversity of twenty-first century globalized societies.

Pandemics are shaped by a multitude of risk factors contributing to the emergence of diverse types of infectious diseases (see Figure 10.1) (World Health Organization 2013). For example, social demographic risk factors like urbanization and rapid population growth strain agricultural and environmental systems, resulting in increased susceptibility to emerging infectious diseases via the effects of variables such as forest clearance, climate change, increased contact with disease vectors, and expanded agricultural activities (World Health Organization 2013; Morse et al. 2012).

Some of the key risk factors for pandemics include: 1) *social risk factors*, such as increases in the hypermobility of persons, urbanization, and exponential population growth (Australian Public Service Commission 2007; Alirol et al. 2011; Bisignani 2011; Duit and Galaz 2008; Hill 2011; Forster 2012; Institute of Medicine 2001; International Air Transport Association 2011; Stephen et al. 2011); 2) *economic risk factors*, such as increases in cross-border trade, changes to food systems, changes in animal-human proximity, and illicit activities like illegal trading of wildlife and exotic pets (World Trade Organization 2010; Smith 2008; Collins and Wall 2004; Macpherson 2005; United States Department of Health and Human Services 2012); and 3) *environmental risk factors*, such as climate changes which alter the way diseases spread and changes in land use (Dean and Fenton 2010; Patz et al. 2004).

Fortunately, many potentially protective factors against the consequences of pandemic emergence have also been identified. These include: 1) *social protective factors*, such as increasing awareness about pandemics and communicating risks to the public, reinforcing public health strategies to prevent pandemic emergence, and developing adequate governance tools and structures for decision-making (Government Accountability Office 2010; Stoto 2012; Ali et al. 2013; Larson 2007; World Health Organization and UNICEF 2009; Bogich et al. 2012; Wilbanks and Kates 1999; McDougall 2010; World Health Organization 2007); 2) *economic protective factors*, such as boosting trade systems and institutions and fighting corruption (World Organization for Animal Health 2013; World Organization for Animal Health 2013b; Asia-Pacific Economic Cooperation, 2007); and 3) *environmental protective factors*, such as designing surveillance programs at the animal-ecosystem interface, preserving balance within ecosystems for the interdependent maintenance of health and biodiversity, and supporting resilience in environments and propensity to adapt to change (FAO, OIE, WHO-UN System Influenza Coordination, UNICEF and The World Bank 2008; Kilpatrick and Randolph 2012; Gunderson and Holling 2001; Forster 2012; Folke, et al., 2005).

Existing Pandemic Plans and Health System Arrangements, Programs and Strategies are Sub-optimal

The second further complicating development is the recognition that existing pandemic plans and health system arrangements, programs and strategies are sub-optimal.

Challenges with Existing Pandemic Plans

The world has greatly advanced its capacity to respond to future global pandemics. In fact, as of 2011, 158 countries around the world had developed pandemic-preparedness plans, most of which were based on anticipating an H5N1 outbreak (World Health Organization 2011b). Despite these advances, it is unclear how

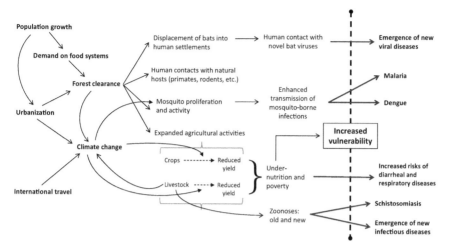

Figure 10.1   Some pandemic risk factors and their relationship to infectious disease emergence

many preparedness plans are actually operational at the country level due to a lack of evaluation, but it is doubtful that all countries have the institutional capacity to implement their plans in a state of emergency (*The Economist* 2013). This is particularly true of many developing countries that lack the capacity to support basic sanitation programs, let alone system-wide pandemic-preparedness systems (Bogich et al. 2012). Thus, while the sheer number of plans and strategies being developed for pandemic response is admirable and important, many are unlikely to be fully implemented.

Further, classical conceptions of global health planning in terms of vertical, disease-specific programs may have undermined basic public health infrastructure and long-term health systems development, potentially diminishing developing countries' health system capacity to respond to future global pandemics (Sridhar 2012). Current plans have failed to fundamentally modify human-environment dynamics at the scale that some experts say are needed, given that plans are focused on post-emergence response rather than prevention (Bogich et al. 2012). Preparedness plans also do not fully address key drivers of pandemic emergence, often lacking diverse strategies to achieve an effective systems approach able to accommodate all of the drivers and actors that could influence pandemic origins, response and recovery in a particular context (Bogich et al. 2012). Calls for comprehensive health system strengthening in recent years have sought to remedy some of these gaps, although full implementation has yet to be observed, particularly in developing countries (Samb et al. 2010).

Although considerable research evidence has recognized the vital role of communities in pandemic response, many pandemic preparedness plans do not currently support participatory epidemiology and other innovative strategies that involve bottom-up, community-based approaches to disease surveillance and management (Wilbanks and Kates 1999; Weinberg 2013; Charania and Tsuji 2012). Despite growing recognition for the role of non-expert citizens as contributors to health system decision-making, the availability of innovative technologies for performing real-time situational analyses during pandemics is limited. For example, Lajous et al.'s (2009) assessment of cellphone technologies as potential surveillance and information dissemination tools during the H1N1 outbreak concluded that 'when carefully deployed, unstructured supplementary service data surveys may be a practical, low-cost, and timely complement to traditional surveillance', yet little mention of mobile technologies exists in today's pandemic preparedness plans. Mobile phone technologies have proven successful in empowering everyday citizens in developing countries to make autonomous choices about HIV/AIDS management, and have been recognized as potentially game-changing tools in improving health crises management (Lester and Karanja 2008).

Additionally, the role of social media in pandemic surveillance and response has not been given full consideration in modern preparedness plans despite recognition for its role in expediting access to information in times of global crises. For instance, the number of followers on the Centers for Disease Control and Prevention's (CDC) Twitter account increased from 2,500 before the H1N1 flu outbreak to 370,000 in late June 2009 (Currie 2009). This suggests the utility of social media to communicate with large numbers of people and the interest among citizens in receiving real-time health information in this way. During H1N1, the CDC used seven kinds of social media tools: buttons and badges, e-Cards, Flickr, Twitter, Facebook, YouTube, widgets and podcasts (Ding and Zhang 2010). Not all pandemic leaders have yet to give serious attention to social media technologies or adopt real-time data collection and surveillance strategies.

Challenges with Existing Delivery Arrangements within Health Systems

Capacity for health systems to take on additional patient loads during pandemics is severely constrained given that institutions are consistently operating at near-maximum efficiency with limited resources (Elharram et al. 2013). Limited laboratory capacity for conducting large-scale rapid diagnostic testing constrains the number of samples that can be examined each day. Moreover, diagnostic surge capacity in laboratories is sometimes inadequate and not supported by appropriate resources and legal frameworks. For example, during an outbreak of H7N3 avian influenza in the Fraser Valley of British Columbia in 2004, the Canadian federal government was only able to confirm results in a laboratory three provinces away, causing an almost 48-hour delay in diagnostic confirmation that may have compromised the effectiveness of pandemic containment strategies (Tweed et al. 2004). During the H1N1 outbreak in Mexico there were also insufficient laboratories for analysis, and those that were present were insufficiently equipped, limiting the quality and diversity of information they could gather (Ear 2011).

Furthermore, community resilience and pandemic prevention infrastructure and resources are difficult to maintain during the inter-pandemic period when the issue is not at the top of the political agenda. It is difficult to justify continued investment in pandemic preparedness given that public health practitioners face significant challenges in measuring the outcomes of successful prevention efforts such as quantifying how many pathogenic agents were prevented from reaching pandemic levels due to effective prevention control programs. Communities also face so many other pressing public health challenges and have so few resources available to act upon them. Moreover, local healthcare delivery systems have often failed to maintain ongoing surveillance, monitoring and evaluation assessments to identify and protect vulnerable communities (Shi and Stevens 2005; Vaughan and Tinker 2009).

Challenges with Existing Financial Arrangements within Health Systems

In federated countries, pandemic governance is challenging when responsibility for health is divided between jurisdictions (Health Canada 2004). For example, in a review of Canada's response to H1N1, it was noted that existing federal financial mechanisms are not sufficiently agile to rapidly support or coordinate activities at the provincial level where health services are primarily funded (Public Health Agency of Canada 2010). Lacking contingency funds from the federal government and the absence of mechanisms to provide urgently needed funding for project proposals precluded the initiation of rapid research projects by sub-national jurisdictions (Public Health Agency of Canada 2010). Additionally, governments in Canada were found to lack standardized processes to rapidly set research priorities during a pandemic and to critically evaluate proposals for research funding against priorities (Public Health Agency of Canada 2010). It is likely that these challenges are faced by other federated jurisdictions too.

During the H1N1 pandemic, many countries also encountered difficulties in equitably allocating funding in a way that reached disadvantaged groups (Public Health Agency of Canada 2010; Ear 2011; Stoto 2012). Funding channels for general care and treatment services can also be particularly inequitable in countries where there is no social health insurance and where many people are uninsured. This problem is compounded by lower rates of health insurance among people with lower incomes. Even as recently as September 2013 and in the world's wealthiest country, 24.9% of Americans in households earning less than $25,000 did not have insurance compared with 15.4% of the entire population, especially problematic given this socioeconomic group also bears a higher burden of disease and comorbidities than wealthier people (Pear 2013).

Challenges with Existing Governance Arrangements within Health Systems

A failure to share information and coordinate actions at the governmental level can impair the process of leading effective responses to pandemic outbreaks. For example, prior to the H1N1 outbreak in Canada, an agreement was developed that included an annex on surveillance information sharing for epidemiologic and laboratory data. While this annex was approved by most jurisdictions, during H1N1 it became apparent that no enforcement mechanisms were in place to ensure processes of transparent information sharing between provinces and the federal government. Although data have been shared previously, there are currently no further commitments to share information in the event of a future pandemic (Public Health Agency of Canada 2010). In Mexico, it was found that loyalty to political parties was detrimental to the effectiveness of the H1N1 response, and that 'in-fighting among the ministries' prevented fluid information sharing between officials (Ear 2011). It has been reported that there was limited coordination at the start of the H1N1 outbreak among Mexico's Ministry of Health, Ministry of Agriculture, Livestock, Rural Development, Fisheries and Food, Ministry of Civil Protection, and Ministry of Defense, resulting in delayed decision-making (Ear 2011).

The timeliness of information sharing can be another obstacle to adopting evidence-based approaches during pandemics, even among high-income countries. For example, during the H1N1 pandemic, the Public Health Agency of Canada experienced challenges with respect to its national surveillance capacity, including both a lack of real-time data on key epidemiological variables and human resources to review surveillance data (Public Health Agency of Canada 2010). In the United States, Stoto (2012) identified a 60-day difference in the release of surveillance data between northeastern states and southern states, reflecting different regional interpretations of risk and abilities to rapidly share information rather than real differences in H1N1 infection rates. Further analysis revealed underlying problems with surveillance systems in the US, particularly their dependence on patient and provider reports (which are influenced by changing information environments) that could limit situational awareness in future public health emergencies (Stoto 2012). In addition, some commentators have pointed to poorly designed consultative processes creating delays in pandemic decision-making and directly interfering with front-line health professionals responding to urgent patient needs (Public Health Agency of Canada 2010).

Finally, a failure to recognize that health is increasingly influenced by decisions that are made in other global policymaking arenas, such as those governing international trade, investment, education, migration and the environment, has impaired some health system responses to pandemic emergence. For example, a lack of formalized legislation granting federal governments unrestricted access to sub-national and sector-specific surveillance data during pandemics has impeded national efforts to coordinate intersectoral action in times of outbreak (Wilson 2006). Limited relationship-building opportunities and irregular communication have also contributed to insufficient trust between authorities from different sectors and jurisdictions, potentially narrowing the range of actors who can help implement a coordinated pandemic response (Axelsson and Axelsson 2006; Willumsen et al. 2012). Health actors today are largely unequipped to ensure their concerns are considered in crucial non-health policymaking arenas, suggesting that opportunities for inclusive approaches to pandemic responses are not being fully exploited (Frenk and Moon 2013).

Challenges with Existing Global Governance Arrangements

Recent experiences with global pandemics have forced the international community to consider whether current global pandemic governance arrangements are adequate. Although the revised IHR were lauded as groundbreaking, in reality, many countries did not meet the June 2012 implementation deadline and have requested a two-year extension to continue scaling-up and measuring national capacity for pandemic preparedness (Ijaz et al. 2012). It has become apparent that many countries do not have adequate research, workforce, laboratory or surveillance capacity to support broad-spectrum pandemic responses. Neither does WHO, which currently has an estimated influenza budget of $7.7 million, an amount equivalent to less than one-third of what the city of New York dedicates to public health emergencies (*The Economist* 2013). It is doubtful that developing countries will be able to fund pandemic preparedness and surveillance schemes on their own.

There have been several promising global initiatives to address this capacity gap, but full implementation has not been achieved. For example, in 2006, WHO aimed to produce enough influenza vaccine to immunize two billion people by 2015, and hoped vaccines would be available on the market 'six months after transfer of the vaccine prototype strain to vaccine manufacturers' during global influenza pandemics. As an indicator of the difficulty in achieving this goal, by December 1, 2009, the six-month milestone for the H1N1 pandemic, global production reached just 534 million doses, and capacity was mostly restricted to the highest-income countries (Partridge and Kieny 2010). Similarly, while there has been significant advocacy for the One Health movement, its operationalization globally has been slow because it requires the coordination of several international institutions and the different government ministries that represent their countries to them (Bogich et al. 2012).

Overall, the conclusion from the 2011 Review Committee on the Functioning of the International Health Regulations (2005) was a sobering reminder that the world is 'ill-prepared to respond to a severe influenza pandemic or to any similarly global, sustained and threatening public-health emergency', and that despite existing arrangements in support of pandemic responses, health systems at all levels are currently inadequately equipped to cope with the burdens of serious pandemics (World Health Organization 2011b).

Approaches to Strengthening Health Systems' Capacity to Respond to Future Global Pandemics

Three approaches to strengthening future responses to global pandemics have been promoted as particularly fruitful: 1) enhancing disease surveillance; 2) preparing for pandemics' variability; and 3) strengthening global pandemic governance. These three approaches were identified based on literature reviews, 12 key informant interviews, and a formal consultation with 18 experts in pandemic preparedness, infectious disease control, epidemiology, risk communications, government policymaking, and related fields, and presented here more as a starting point for analysis than as a conclusive statement about priorities.

We reviewed available research evidence about each of these three identified approaches.[1] While some of the research evidence may not deal specifically with pandemics, we included it when it could provide relevant insights and spur reflection about each approach. Our focus was on what is known about these approaches based on findings from systematic reviews as well as economic evaluations or costing studies. We present the findings from systematic reviews along with an appraisal using the AMSTAR tool of whether their methodological quality is high (scores of 8 or higher out of 11), medium (scores of 4 to 7) or low (scores below 4) (Shea et al. 2007).

Approach #1: Enhancing Disease Surveillance

The first approach involves enhancing national health systems' disease surveillance capacity, such as detecting pandemic risk factors, identifying causal pathogens, characterizing emerging diseases, and monitoring their evolution. Elements of this approach include:

1. Enhancing ongoing surveillance systems' capacity to detect, identify and investigate emergence risk factors and early disease outbreaks, and

---

1   The available research evidence about approaches for addressing the problem was sought primarily from Health Systems Evidence (www.healthsystemsevidence.org), which is a continuously updated database containing more than 3,000 systematic reviews and more than 1,600 economic evaluations of delivery, financial and governance arrangements within health systems. The reviews were identified by searching the database for records addressing features of each of the approaches and elements. The authors' conclusions were extracted from the reviews whenever possible. Some reviews contained no studies despite an exhaustive search, while others concluded that there was substantial uncertainty about the approach based on the identified studies. Where relevant, caveats were introduced about these authors' conclusions based on assessments of the reviews' quality, the local applicability of the reviews' findings, equity considerations, and relevance to the issue. No additional research evidence about the approaches was sought beyond what was included in the systematic reviews.

effectively monitor the evolution of disease such as its epidemiology, clinical manifestations, severity and rate of transmission;

2. Integrating top-down surveillance programs with bottom-up approaches for monitoring and mitigating risks and overcoming current legal barriers for sharing information gathered across sectors and ministries;
3. Building capacity for rapid data collection, analysis and assessment by decision-makers across jurisdictions through enhanced information and communication technologies such as platforms that would allow various authorities to access real-time national diagnostic data;
4. Providing dedicated funding for knowledge management and monitoring systems;
5. Working to improve global surveillance, outbreak management and investigation systems, especially in low-income and high-risk countries; and
6. Establishing collaborative interprofessional teams to conduct routine surveillance, particularly for zoonotic disease outbreaks, that enhance human and animal surveillance system linkages.

We found five high-quality systematic reviews pointing to the benefits of enhancing ongoing surveillance systems' capacity (element 1) (Leal and Laupland 2008), building capacity for shared rapid data collection, analysis and assessment (element 3) (Lobach et al. 2012; Lau et al. 2010), and establishing collaborative interprofessional teams to conduct routine surveillance (element 6) (Medves et al. 2010; Barrett et al. 2007). These reviews provide good evidence for pursuing policies and programs that would leverage these elements. We were unable to identify any systematic reviews to inform integrating top-down surveillance programs with bottom-up approaches for monitoring risks (element 1.2), providing dedicated funding for knowledge management and information and monitoring systems (element 1.4), or working to improve global surveillance, outbreak management and investigation systems (element 1.5). This does not mean these elements are not worth pursuing, but it does indicate that further research is needed to confirm whether these elements would generate benefits or potential harms. Monitoring and evaluation could be warranted if the option were pursued.

Approach #2: Preparing for Pandemics' Variability

The second approach involves strengthening the capacity of national policymakers, stakeholders and the public to respond to the variability of pandemics that could be encountered. Elements of this approach include:

1. Enhancing relationship-building, learning, trust and transfer of knowledge from researchers to policymakers via ongoing communications during pre-, inter- and post-pandemic periods;
2. Implementing adaptive governance structures that enable policymakers and stakeholders to respond to the variability of pandemics and which

assist decision-makers in navigating the complex informational landscape that frequently evolves during a pandemic;

3. Developing a health risk communication strategy to help politicians and the public become aware of, prepare for, and adapt to the emerging threat of a pandemic, and which strengthens communication among national, sub-national, global and non-state actors to ensure the efficient and transparent sharing of accurate information;

4. Establishing well-recognized authorities as trusted sources of information that can lead communication efforts with the public during pandemics and who are equipped to communicate complex information to people with low levels of health literacy; and

5. Developing methods to utilize mobile phones, crowd-sourcing technologies and popular social media tools such as Facebook, Twitter and LinkedIn for both disease surveillance and risk communication.

Nine medium- and high-quality systematic reviews found benefits for key elements of this approach, including information products designed to support the uptake of systematic review evidence (element 1) (Murthy et al. 2012), public engagement to inform policymaking (element 2.2) (Conklin et al. 2012; Abelson et al. 2010; Menon et al. 2003), risk communication strategies (element 2.3) (Campbell et al. 2009), and mobile phone text messages (element 2.5) (Car et al. 2012; Horvath et al. 2012; Wei et al. 2011). The findings of these reviews indicates that implementation of any of elements 2.1–2.3 and 2.5 would strengthen systems' capacity to respond to the variability of pandemics, and should be given serious consideration by decision-makers leading efforts in this area.

Approach #3: Strengthening Global Pandemic Governance

The third approach involves strengthening the global pandemic governance system, which is the broader context within which national health systems' responses would be implemented. It empowers and constrains actions. Possible changes to the global pandemic governance system include better communication, collaboration and policy coherence among national governments and international agencies. Elements of this approach might include:

1. Establishing more effective mechanisms of global coordination and policy coherence to better manage trans-border trade and other economic activities during pandemics;

2. Identifying what kinds of legal and policy responses should be taken to correct a failure of cooperation on the part of governments within states and at the national level;

3. Developing mechanisms to support international dispute resolution, plus developing effective enforcement mechanisms, and/or incentives to support national compliance with international regulations and other obligations;

4. Creating more flexibility and responsiveness within the global system to collectively adapt to uncertainty, such as by developing priority-setting procedures, better coordinating responsibilities between countries, and having technical assistance ready for those who need it;
5. Improving WHO's information dissemination process to stakeholders and Member States, including enhancement of WHO's Event Information Site; and
6. Supporting health systems capacity-building in high-risk developing countries to respond to future pandemics as per developed countries' international legal responsibilities to provide support to developing countries under the IHR.

We found little synthesized research evidence that can be drawn upon to inform the elements of this approach. Four systematic reviews speak to some benefits for elements 3.1 and 3.6, more specifically, global health initiatives for HIV/AIDS control (Biesma et al. 2009), contracting out healthcare services in developing countries (Lagarde and Palmer 2009), result-based financing (Oxman and Fretheim 2008), and developing international nursing curricula through cooperative partnerships (Sochan 2008). We found no systematic reviews relevant to the other four elements which means monitoring and evaluation are essential should they be implemented.

Prioritizing Elements of the Three Approaches with the Greatest Potential Benefit

Of the various approaches and elements that were identified in our literature reviews, key informant interviews and formal consultation, we found the strongest evidence supporting:

- Enhancing ongoing surveillance systems' capacity (element 1.1);
- Building capacity for shared rapid data collection, analysis and assessment (element 1.3);
- Establishing collaborative interprofessional teams to conduct routine surveillance (element 1.6);
- Developing information products designed to support the uptake of systematic review evidence (element 2.1);
- Supporting public engagement to inform policymaking (element 2.2);
- Designing risk communication strategies (element 2.3);
- Capitalizing on mobile phone text messaging as a tool to effectively capture situational analyses within pandemic management (element 2.5);
- Supporting global governance and coordination systems for health and trade, particularly given the evidence from global health initiatives for HIV/AIDS control (element 3.1); and

- Developing health systems capacity in high-risk developing countries to detect, diagnose, respond to, and communicate situations of pandemic emergence (element 3.6).

This does not mean these particular strategies will necessarily have the greatest positive effects, but it does mean that there is more synthesized research evidence suggesting benefit and guiding implementation efforts than for the other strategies.

Implementation Considerations

Although this chapter has presented three approaches to addressing the challenge of strengthening pandemic responses, obstacles to implementation could undermine efforts for change. All of the challenges posed by pandemics cannot just be solved if decision-makers had better tools, more money, or new legislation. Rather, they need to be effectively employed at the right level and in the right way for whatever political, social and economic contexts are faced. It is not possible to define the desired state of preparedness in technical terms for every context, but optimal readiness might, for example, balance affordability, feasibility and adequate protection. With those underlying goals in mind, it is possible to begin to assess the importance of barriers to implementation and set priorities for action.

Potential Barriers to Implementing the Three Approaches

Sub-national policymakers may be hesitant to adopt new information and communication technology or reporting protocols, and may be reluctant to spend the money and time required to re-train health personnel to adopt the new surveillance measures called for in approach #1. With respect to approach #2, the ability for officials to communicate risk through the media may be compromised in some areas, and policymakers may find it difficult to develop flexible, adaptive emergence-management structures across jurisdictions. In trying to strengthen the global pandemic governance system, approach #3 may encounter resistance from sub-national policymakers hesitant to let national or global governing bodies dictate priorities during pandemic outbreaks from afar.

National policymakers may struggle to convince their sub-national counterparts to openly share their surveillance data with other jurisdictions when trying to implement approach #1. It may be challenging to implement approach #2 given how sub-national governments may prefer to lead on risk communications with their constituents. It may be challenging for federal decision-makers to implement approach #3 given that policymakers from sub-national jurisdictions may resist the federal government adopting a formal information-sharing agreement with other countries.

At the global level, member states of multilateral organizations may hold conflicting opinions over what constitutes best evidence in decision-making, making it difficult to reach the global consensus noted in approach #1, particularly if they choose to unilaterally act in opposition to an integrated approach with other countries. It may be challenging to implement approach #2 if countries are restricted from contributing to, or receiving information from, a global platform for information sharing because of their limited infrastructural and resource capacities. For approach #3, implementation could be compromised by collective action problems and unwillingness to receiving criticism about response strategies as can be issued by WHO under the IHR.

Some implementation barriers are faced at all levels of governance. For example, securing sustained, long-term financing for public health infrastructure and integrated approaches to pandemic preparedness, particularly during the pre- and inter-pandemic periods, may prevent policymakers at every level from acting on any of the three approaches even if they strongly wish to do so.

Potential Windows of Opportunity for Implementing the Approaches

Despite the potential barriers to action outlined above, there are several windows of opportunity that could facilitate positive change. For instance, the sobering findings of WHO's 2011 IHR Review concluded that the world is still underprepared to adequately manage the next severe pandemic threat or other serious public health emergency, which could help motivate policymakers at all levels to enhance current efforts for pandemic preparedness. In fact, the review called for increased preparedness through research, strengthened health systems and multi-sectoral approaches (World Health Organization 2011b). That same year, WHO adopted a Pandemic Influenza Preparedness Framework that balances the need for virus sharing and access to vaccines developed with these shared viruses (World Health Organization 2011). The Harvard Business Review and World Economic Forum have named global pandemics as one of the top 'megatrends' and 'risks' facing the world, acknowledging how urban sprawl, population growth, global travel, and rudimentary health systems in poorer countries ensure this threat remains serious (Dillon and Prokesch 2011; World Economic Forum 2013).

Recent efforts have also been launched at the regional level to evaluate and scale up pandemic response capacity. For example, a report by Trust for America's Health and the Robert Wood Johnson Foundation (2013) identified major gaps in the US' ability to prevent, control, and respond to infectious disease threats due to outdated systems and limited resources. The report revealed that the majority of states ($n=32$) scored 5 or lower out of 10 key indicators of policies and capabilities to protect against infectious disease outbreaks. The report called for renewed governmental action and 'cooperative efforts with the healthcare sector; pharmaceutical, medical supply and technology companies; community groups, schools and employers; and families and individuals' to secure every American's 'right to basic protections no matter where they live' (Trust for America's Health and The Robert Wood Johnson Foundation 2013: 4). In April 2012, a new North American Plan for Animal and Pandemic Influenza (NAPAPI) was announced at that year's North American Leaders Summit attended by heads of government in

Washington, D.C. The plan calls for action to further strengthen the continental response to future global animal and pandemic influenzas (Public Health Agency of Canada 2012). In 2011, the Association of Southeast Asian Nations launched a five-year pandemic preparedness plan that includes critical sectors like food, energy, water, sanitation, telecommunications, finance, public security, justice, transportation, and health (Association of Southeast Asian Nations Secretariat 2011). Additionally, efforts have been underway at global inter-ministerial meetings on animal and human influenza in 2007, 2009 and 2010, to enhance the uptake of One Health models in the surveillance of zoonotic disease emergence (American Veterinary Association 2008).

Ongoing media coverage of the Middle East respiratory syndrome (MERS) and avian influenza H7N9 outbreaks in Saudi Arabia and China, respectively, highlight that pandemics loom on the cusp of emergence. Public calls for increased government transparency and capacity-building have given pandemic preparedness greater political prioritization on the global agenda (Harada et al. 2013). In May 2013, WHO Director-General Margaret Chan opened her speech to the 66th World Health Assembly on the subject of pandemics, citing the novel coronavirus in the Eastern Mediterranean region and France, and the H7N9 avian influenza virus in China. In her words: 'These two new diseases remind us that the threat from emerging and epidemic-prone diseases is ever-present. Constant mutation and adaptation are the survival mechanisms of the microbial world. It will always deliver surprises.' Chan called for vigilance, transparency in reporting, collaboration and cooperation for pandemic preparedness, and adherence to the IHR (Chan 2013).

Conclusion

The threat posed by global pandemics necessitates further efforts to strengthen national health systems' capacity to respond to them. We have examined the challenges posed by pandemics and provided analysis of three approaches to address them at the sub-national, national and global levels. We have also identified key implementation considerations, including barriers to be overcome and potential windows of opportunity to make substantial gains. None of the approaches can be achieved by any one decision-maker, sector, government or country alone. It is imperative that the world embrace a truly collaborative approach to pandemic preparedness planning so that the profound interconnectedness and interdependence of populations in the twenty-first century is revered as an era of opportunity rather than one of risk and ruin.

Acknowledgments

The authors wish to thank our colleagues from the McMaster Health Forum, John N. Lavis and François-Pierre Gauvin, who co-authored with us an issue brief that inspired this chapter. The authors also thank the Global Health Research Initiative – a research funding partnership composed of the Canadian Institutes of Health Research, Department of Foreign Affairs, Trade and Development, and Canada's International Development Research Centre – for funding these efforts. SJH is financially supported by the Canadian Institutes of Health Research and the Trudeau Foundation.

References

Abelson, J., Montesanti, S., Li, K., et al., 2010. *Effective Strategies for Interactive Public Engagement in the Development of Healthcare Policies and Programs.* Ottawa: Canadian Health Services Research Foundation.

Ali, M., Caroti, A. and Mellor, K., 2013. *Issue Brief: Pandemic Preparedness and the Media – Building Capacity to Improve Communications During Pandemics.* Hamilton, ON: McMaster University.

Alirol, E., Getaz, L., Stoll, B., et al., 2011. Urbanisation and infectious diseases in a globalised world. *Lancet Infectious Diseases*, 11(2): 131–41.

American Veterinary Medical Association, 2008. *One Health: A New Professional Imperative.* Schaumburg, Illinois.: One Health Initiative Task Force.

Asia-Pacific Economic Cooperation, 2007. *Functioning Economies in Times of Pandemic: APEC Guidelines.* Sydney: Asia-Pacific Economic Cooperation.

Association of Southeast Asian Nations (ASEAN) Secretariat, 2011. ASEAN Embarks on New Pandemic Preparedness Plan. *ASEAN Secretariat News.* Available at: http://www.asean.org/news/asean-secretariat-news/item/asean-embarks-on-new-pandemic-preparedness-plan [Accessed 14 December 2013].

Australian Public Service Commission, 2007. *Tackling Wicked Problems: A Public Policy Perspective.* Barton, Australia: Australian Public Service Commission.

Axelsson, R. and Axelsson, S.B., 2006. Integration and collaboration in public health – A conceptual framework. *International Journal of Health Planning and Management*, 21(1): 75–88.

Barrett, J., Curran, V., Glynn, L. and Godwin, M., 2007. *Interprofessional Collaboration and Quality Primary Healthcare.* Ottawa: Canadian Health Services Research Foundation.

Bechard, N., Hoit, G. and Pullen, N., 2013. *Issue Brief: Pandemic Preparedness from the Perspective of Multilateral Organizations and National Partnerships.* Hamilton, ON: McMaster University.

Biesma, R.G., Brugha, R., Harmer, A., et al., 2009. The effects of global health initiatives on country health systems: A review of the evidence from HIV/AIDS control. *Health Policy and Planning*, 24(4): 239–52.

Bisignani, G., 2011. *Remarks of Giovanni Bisignani at the Vision 2050 press briefing, Singapore.* International Air Transport Association. Available at: http://www.iata.org/pressroom/speeches/Pages/2011-02-14-01.aspx [Accessed 15 September 2013].

Bogich, T.L., Chunara, R., Scales, D., et al., 2012. Preventing pandemics via international development: A systems approach. *PLoS Medicine,* 9(12), p.e1001354.

Campbell, M., Buckeridge, D., Dwyer, J., et al., 2009. A systematic review of the effectiveness of environmental awareness interventions. *Canadian Journal of Public Health,* 91(2): 137–43.

Car, J., Gurol-Urganci, I., de, J.T., Vodopivec-Jamsek, V., Atun, R., 2012. Mobile phone messaging reminders for attendance at healthcare appointments. *Cochrane Database of Systematic Reviews,* 7, p.CD007458.

Chan, M., 2013. *WHO Director-General addresses the sixty-sixth World Health Assembly.* Geneva: World Health Organization.

Charania, N.A. and Tsuji, L.J., 2012. A community-based participatory approach and engagement process creates culturally appropriate and community informed pandemic plans after the 2009 H1N1 influenza pandemic: Remote and isolated First Nations communities of sub-arctic Ontario, Canada. *BMC Public Health,* 12: 268.

Cole-Lewis, H. and Kershaw, T., 2010. Text messaging as a tool for behavior change in disease prevention and management. *Epidemiolic Review,* 32(1): 56–69.

Collins, J.D. and Wall, P.G., 2004. Food safety and animal production systems: Controlling zoonoses at farm level. *Revue Scientifique et Technique,* 23(2): 685–700.

Conklin, A., Morris, Z. and Nolte, E., 2012. *What is the evidence base for public involvement in health-care policy? Results of a systematic scoping review.* Health Expectations.

Currie, D., 2009. Public health turning to social media to communicate risks. *The Nation's Health,* pp. 9–10.

Day, J., 2013. *Pandemic Controversies: The Global Response to Pandemic Influenza Must Change.* Brighton: STEPS Centre.

Dean, H. and Fenton, K., 2010. Addressing social determinants of health in the prevention and control of HIV/AIDS, viral hepatitis, sexually transmitted infections and tuberculosis. *Public Health Reports,* 125(4): 1–5.

Del Rio, C. and Hernandez-Avila, M., 2009. Lessons from previous influenza pandemics and from the Mexican response to the current influenza pandemic. *Archives of Medical Research,* 40(8): 677–80.

Dillon, K. and Prokesch, S., 2011. Megatrends in Global Health Care. *Harvard Business Review.* Available at: http://hbr.org/web/extras/insight-center/health-care/globaltrends/1-slide [Accessed 4 September 2013].

Ding, H. and Zhang, J., 2010. Social media and participatory risk communication during the H1N1 flue epidemic: A comparative study of the United States and China. *China Media Research,* 6(4): 80–91.

Duit, A. and Galaz, V., 2008. Governance and complexity – Emerging issues for governance theory. *Governance*, 21(3): 311–35.

Ear, S., 2011. *Towards Effective Emerging Infectious Disease Surveillance: H1N1 in the United States 1976 and Mexico 2009.* Munich: University Library of Munich.

Economist, The, 2013. Coming, Ready Or Not: Despite Progress, the World is Still Unprepared for a New Pandemic Disease. *The Economist*. Available at: http://www.economist.com/news/leaders/21576390-despite-progress-world-still-unprepared-new-pandemic-disease-coming-ready-or-not [Accessed 10 November 2013].

Elharram, M., Jedrzejko, N., Lau, K. and Vignesh, N., 2013. *Issue Brief: Addressing Pandemic Preparedness Issues within Local Healthcare Institutions.* Hamilton, ON: McMaster University.

FAO, OIE, WHO-UN System Influenza Coordination, UNICEF, The World Bank, 2008. *Contributing to One World, One Health – A Strategic Framework for Reducing Risks of Infectious Diseases at the Animal-Human-Ecosystems Interface.* Food and Agriculture Organization of the United Nations. Available at: http://www.fao.org/docrep/011/aj137e/aj137e00.htm [Accessed 10 November 2013].

Folke, C., Hahn, T., Olsson, P. and Norberg, J., 2005. Adaptive governance of social-ecological systems. *Annual Review of Environmental Resources*, 30(1): 441–73.

Forster, P., 2012. *To Pandemic or Not? Reconfiguring Global Responses to Influenza.* Brighton: STEPS Centre.

Frenk, J. and Moon, S., 2013. Governance challenges in global health. *New England Journal of Medicine*, 368(10): 936–42.

Government Accountability Office, 2010. *Public Health Information Technology: Additional Strategic Planning Needed to Guide HHS's Efforts to Establish Electronic Situational Awareness Capabilities.* Washington, DC: Government Accountability Office.

Gunderson, L. and Holling, C., 2001. *Panarchy: Understanding Transformations in Human and Natural Systems.* Washington, DC: Island Press.

Harada, N., Alexander, N. and Olowokure, B., 2013. Avian influenza A(H7N9): Information-sharing through government web sites in the Western Pacific Region. *Western Pacific Surveillance and Response Journal*, 4(2): 44–6.

Health Canada, 2004. *Health Care System: Federal Role in Health Care.* Health Canada. Available at: http://www.hc-sc.gc.ca/hcs-sss/delivery-prestation/fedrole/index-eng.php [Accessed 26 September 2013].

Hill, P.S., 2011. Understanding global health governance as a complex adaptive system. *Global Public Health*, 6(6): 593–605.

Hoffman, S.J., 2010. The evolution, etiology and eventualities of the global health security regime. *Health Policy and Planning*, 25(6): 510–22.

Horvath, T., Azman, H., Kennedy, G.E., Rutherford, G.W., 2012. Mobile phone text messaging for promoting adherence to antiretroviral therapy in patients with HIV infection. *Cochrane Database of Systematic Reviews*, 3, p.CD009756.

Ijaz, K., Kasowski, E., Arthur, R.R., et al., 2012. International Health Regulations – What gets measured gets done. *Emerging Infectious Diseases*, 18(7): 1054–7.

Institute of Medicine, 2001. *Crossing the Quality Chasm: A New Health System for the 21st Century*. Washington, DC: Institute of Medicine.

International Air Transport Association, 2011. *Successful Vision 2050 Meeting Concludes – Building a Sustainable Future*. International Air Transport Association. Available at: http://www.iata.org/pressroom/pr/Pages/2011-02-14-01.aspx [Accessed 15 September 2013].

Johnson, N.P. and Mueller, J., 2002. Updating the accounts: Global mortality of the 1918–1920 'Spanish' influenza pandemic. *Bulletin of the History of Medicine*, 76(1): 105–15.

Kamradt-Scott, A., 2011. The evolving WHO: Implications for global health security. *Global Public Health*, 6(8): 801–13.

Kilpatrick, A.M. and Randolph, S.E., 2012. Drivers, dynamics, and control of emerging vector-borne zoonotic diseases. *Lancet*, 380(9857): 1946–55.

Lagarde, M. and Palmer, N., 2009. The impact of contracting out on health outcomes and use of health services in low and middle-income countries. *Cochrane Database of Systematic Reviews*, 4, p.CD008133.

Lajous, M., Danon, L., Lopez-Ridaura, R., et al., 2010. Mobile messaging as surveillance tool during pandemic (H1N1) 2009, Mexico. *Emerging Infectious Diseases*, 16(9): 1488–9.

Larson, E., 2007. Community factors in the development of antibiotic resistance. *Annual Review of Public Health*, 28: 435–47.

Lau, F., Kuziemsky, C., Price, M., Gardner, J., 2010. A review on systematic reviews of health information system studies. *Journal of the American Medical Informatics Association*, 17(6): 637–45.

Leal, J. and Laupland, K.B., 2008. Validity of electronic surveillance systems: A systematic review. *Journal of Hospital Infection*, 69(3): 220–29.

Lee, K. and Fidler, D., 2007. Avian and pandemic influenza: Progress and problems with global health governance. *Global Public Health*, 2(3): 215–34.

Lester, R. and Karanja, S., 2008. Mobile phones: Exceptional tools for HIV/AIDS, health, and crisis management. *Lancet Infectious Diseases*, 8(12): 738–9.

Lobach, D., Sanders, G.D., Bright, T.J., et al., 2012. Enabling health care decisionmaking through clinical decision support and knowledge management. *Evidence Report/Technology Assessment*, 203: 1–784.

Macpherson, C.N., 2005. Human behaviour and the epidemiology of parasitic zoonoses. *International Journal of Parasitology*, 35(11–12): 1319–31.

McDougall, C., 2010. *A Survey of Ethical Principles and Guidance Within Selected Pandemic Plans*. Montreal: National Collaborating Centre for Health Public Policy, Institut national de santé publique du Québec.

Medves, J., Godfrey, C., Turner, C., et al., 2010. Systematic review of practice guideline dissemination and implementation strategies for healthcare teams and team-based practice. *International Journal of Evidence-Based Healthcare*, 8(2): 79–89.

Menon, D., Stafinski, T., Martin, D., et al. 2003. *State of the Science Review: Incorporating Public Values and Technical Information into Health Care Resource Allocation Decision-Making*. Edmonton: Alberta Innovates Health Solutions.

Morse, S.S., Mazet, J.A., Woolhouse, M., et al., 2012. Prediction and prevention of the next pandemic zoonosis. *Lancet*, 380(9857): 1956–65.

Murthy, L., Shepperd, S., Clarke, M.J., et al., 2012. Interventions to improve the use of systematic reviews in decision-making by health system managers, policy makers and clinicians. *Cochrane Database of Systematic Reviews*, 9, p.CD009401.

Office of the Provincial Health Officer of British Columbia, 2010. *Response to the H1N1 Pandemic: A Summary Report*. Vancouver: Office of the Provincial Health Officer.

Oxman, A.D. and Fretheim, A., 2008. *An Overview of Research on the Effects of Results-Based Financing*. Oslo: Norwegian Knowledge Centre for the Health Services.

Partridge, J. and Kieny, M.P., 2010. Global production of seasonal and pandemic (H1N1) influenza vaccines in 2009–2010 and comparison with previous estimates and global action plan targets. *Vaccine*, 28(30): 4709–12.

Patz, J.A., Daszak, P., Tabor, G.M., et al., 2004. Unhealthy landscapes: Policy recommendations on land use change and infectious disease emergence. *Environmental Health Perspectives*, 112(10): 1092–8.

Pear, R., 2013. Percentage of Americans Lacking Health Coverage Falls Again. *The New York Times*. Available at: http://www.nytimes.com/2013/09/18/us/percentage-of-americans-lacking-health-coverage-falls-again.html [Accessed 20 September 2013].

Public Health Agency of Canada, 2010. *Lessons Learned Review: Public Health Agency of Canada and Health Canada Response to the 2009 H1N1 Pandemic*. Ottawa: Public Health Agency of Canada.

Public Health Agency of Canada, 2012. *North American Leaders announce revised North American Plan for Animal and Pandemic Influenza (NAPAPI)*. Ottawa: Public Health Agency of Canada. Available at: http://www.phac-aspc.gc.ca/influenza/napinfluenza-eng.php [Accessed 12 September 2013].

Salaam-Blyther, T., 2009. *The 2009 Influenza Pandemic: U.S. Responses to Global Human Cases*. Washington, DC: Congressional Research Service, Library of Congress.

Samb, B., Desai, N., Nishtar, S., et al., 2010. Prevention and management of chronic disease: A litmus test for health-systems strengthening in low-income and middle-income countries. *Lancet*, 376(9754): 1785–97.

Shea, B.J., Grimshaw, J.M., Wells, G.A., et al., 2007. Development of AMSTAR: A measurement tool to assess the methodological quality of systematic reviews. *BMC Medical Research Methodology*, 7: 10.

Shi, L. and Stevens, G.D., 2005. Vulnerability and unmet health care needs: The influence of multiple risk factors. *Journal of General Internal Medicine*, 20(2): 148–54.

Smith, R.D., 2008. *Global Change and Health: Mapping the Challenges of Global Non-Healthcare Influences on Health.* Geneva: World Health Organization.

Sochan, A., 2008. Relationship building through the development of international nursing curricula: A literature review. *International Nursing Review*, 55(2): 192–204.

Sridhar, D., 2012. Who sets the global health research agenda? The challenge of multi-bi financing. *PLoS Medicine*, 9(9), p.e1001312.

Steel-Fisher, G.K., Blendon, R.J., Bekheit, et al., 2010. The public's response to the 2009 H1N1 influenza pandemic. *The New England Journal of Medicine*, 362(22): e65.

Stephen, C., Ninghui, L., Yeh, F. and Zhang, L., 2011. Animal health policy principles for highly pathogenic avian influenza: Shared experience from China and Canada. *Zoonoses Public Health*, 58(5): 334–42.

Stoto, M.A., 2012. The effectiveness of U.S. public health surveillance systems for situational awareness during the 2009 H1N1 pandemic: A retrospective analysis. *PLoS One*, 7(8), p.e40984.

Taubenberger, J.K. and Morens, D.M., 2006. 1918 Influenza: The mother of all pandemics. *Emerging Infectious Diseases*, 12(1): 15–22.

Toner, E., Waldhorn, R., Maldin, B., et al., 2006. Hospital preparedness for pandemic influenza. *Biosecurity and Bioterrorism*, 4(2): 207–17.

Trust for America's Health and The Robert Wood Johnson Foundation, 2013. *Outbreaks: Protecting Americans from Infectious Diseases.* Available at: http://www.rwjf.org/content/dam/farm/reports/reports/2013/rwjf409564 [Accessed 21 January 2014].

Tweed, S.A., Skowronski, D.M., David, S.T., et al., 2004. Human illness from avian influenza H7N3, British Columbia. *Emerging Infectious Diseases*, 10(12): 2196–9.

United States Department of Health and Human Services, 2012. *The North American Plan for Animal and Pandemic Influenza.* Washington, DC: Office of the Assistant Secretary for Preparedness and Response.

Vaughan, E. and Tinker, T., 2009. Effective health risk communication about pandemic influenza for vulnerable populations. *American Journal of Public Health*, 99(Suppl 2): S324-S332.

Wei, J., Hollin, I. and Kachnowski, S., 2011. A review of the use of mobile phone text messaging in clinical and healthy behaviour interventions. *Journal of Telemedicine and Telecare*, 17(1): 41–8.

Weinberg, L., 2013. *Risk Communications in Action on H1N1.* Ogilvy Public Relations. Available at: http://www.ogilvypr.com/en/expert-view/expert-view/risk-communications-action-h1n1 [Accessed 28 September 2013].

Wilbanks, T.J. and Kates, R.W., 1999. Global change in local places: How scale matters. *Climatic Change*, 43(3): 601–28.

Willumsen, E., Ahgren, B. and Odegard, A., 2012. A conceptual framework for assessing interorganizational integration and interprofessional collaboration. *Journal of Interprofessional Care*, 26(3): 198–204.

Wilson, K., 2006. Pandemic threats and the need for new emergency public health legislation in Canada. *Healthcare Policy*, 2(2): 35–42.

Wong, G., 2013. H7N9 is One Of 'Most Lethal' Flu Viruses So Far, WHO Says. *Huffington Post*. Available at: http://www.huffingtonpost.com/2013/04/24/h7 n9-lethal-bird-flu-china-_n_3147043.html [Accessed 5 November 2013].

World Economic Forum, 2013. *Global Risks 2013: Eighth Edition.* Geneva: World Economic Forum. Available at: http://www3.weforum.org/docs/WEF_ GlobalRisks_Report_2013.pdf [Accessed 15 December 2013].

World Health Organization, 2007a. *Ethical Considerations in Developing a Public Health Response to Pandemic Influenza.* Geneva: World Health Organization.

World Health Organization, 2007b. *World Health Report 2007: A Safer Future: Global Public Health Security in the 21st Century.* Available at: http://www. who.int/whr/2007/en/ [Accessed 3 November 2013].

World Health Organization, 2011a. *Pandemic Influenza Preparedness Framework for the Sharing of Influenza Viruses and Access to Vaccines and Other Benefits.* Geneva: World Health Organization.

World Health Organization, 2011b. *Report by the Director-General – Implementation of the International Health Regulations (2005): Report of the Review Committee on the Functioning of the International Health Regulations (2005) in relation to Pandemic (H1N1) 2009.* A64/10 ed. Geneva: World Health Organization.

World Health Organization, 2013. *Research Priorities for the Environment, Agriculture and Infectious Diseases of Poverty.* Geneva: World Health Organization.

World Health Organization and UNICEF, 2009. *Global Action Plan for Prevention and Control of Pneumonia (GAPP).* Geneva: World Health Organization.

World Organization for Animal Health, 2013a. *Aquatic Animal Health Code.* Paris: World Organization for Animal Health.

World Organization for Animal Health, 2013b. *Terrestrial Animal Health Code.* Paris: World Organization for Animal Health.

World Trade Organization, 2010. *World Trade 2009, Prospects for 2010.* Geneva: World Trade Organization.

Zoutman, D.E., Ford, B.D., Melinyshyn, M. and Schwartz, B., 2010. The pandemic influenza planning process in Ontario acute care hospitals. *American Journal of Infection Control*, 38(1): 3–8.

Conclusion

Sara E. Davies and Jeremy R. Youde

In the Introduction of this book we outlined our approach to the topic "politics of disease surveillance" as a statement and a question. Global cooperation in the area of infectious disease surveillance has grown in both the technology and the actors available to assist these programmes. However, as this book demonstrates, access to the technology that informs global surveillance and the actions required to follow up on global surveillance is inherently political. Surveillance is primarily approached and understood as a public health service, but it is also a political act with implications in terms of human rights, governance, resource distribution and cooperation amongst countries.

In addressing the political impact and influence of surveillance technology, the risk assessment and behaviors that flow from this technology requires a deeper chronicle of its political impact, according to different outbreak cases and different regions—to ensure maximum benefit with minimum harm.

Why has surveillance—particularly global surveillance—been appreciated as a benign act until now? Partly, as all the chapters refer, the revised IHR formally recognized the right of the WHO to use these networks to request outbreak information from states. The revised IHR, for the first time in its history, has allowed surveillance conducted by actors other than the state to, potentially, have influence on the action and behavior of both states and the WHO. This is unprecedented, and it leads to a volume of questions about the political and logistical cost of investment in surveillance investment (chapters 1 and 2, chapters 9 and 10); who is culpable when surveillance reports risk but it is ignored or challenged (chapters 3 and 4; chapters 7 and 8); whose surveillance should be trusted (states or non-state actors, as chapters 5 and 6 outlined); and what role do individuals have in determining the extent to which their biodata should be part of a global response to disease outbreaks (Chapter 1). As we saw in all of these chapters, there are different appreciations of how all actors are progressing and failing when it comes to the responses that develop during and after outbreak events.

What is clear is that the political tensions that arise from this technology are as great as its power to minimize tensions. As chapters 2 and 8 highlighted in the cases of H5N1 and H1N1, this technology directs a lens into the actions and behaviors of states that is unprecedented. Outbreaks in remote locations in Sumatra, Indonesia, become global news in a couple of days due to the increased normalization of disease outbreak reporting via social media and traditional media, post SARS. On the other hand, SARS opened up the opportunity for genuine engagement in the need to normalize outbreak events. Ideally, such a shift can ensure more transparency and cooperation in outbreak alerts and response, reduce panic, increase resilience, and increase state cooperation.

In the Introduction, we highlighted five principles—transparency, local engagement, responsiveness to individual needs, integrated operations, and the opportunity to appeal—vital for understanding how, for whom, and to what end global surveillance works. What lessons can we learn from the preceding chapters about those principles?

First, we outlined the need for transparency in both the surveillance process and actions that inform behavior on news of an alert to ensure trust in the technology and the actors that must cooperate in detecting and containing an outbreak. There is, to some extent, greater opportunity for transparency at the global surveillance level than within states. As Chapter 1 discussed, the internet surveillance programme providers—for the most part—are independent. While GPHIN (Chapter 5) is less so than BioCaster (Chapter 6), all of these surveillance providers facilitate locating outbreak event knowledge and highlighting where gaps remain. Just through the daily production of events for each region, we can start to see who is performing and who must not be due to the "surveillance silence." However, such an emphasis on states developing surveillance technology could, counterfactually, compromise their obligation to transparent action. A greater capacity to control and monitor social media and conventional media exchanges could lead governments to act in ways to limit information sharing, but plausibly justify these actions as control mechanisms that allow for one consistent message to be communicated to the public. In most instances this action would be open to scrutiny and condemnation, but as chapters 4 and 8 highlighted, there remains the risk that an emphasis on surveillance alone as the first point of outbreak control justifies the isolation of individuals and, in extreme cases, the introduction of a state of emergency to control what may be reported outside of the state. Moreover, as both chapters 7 and 10 noted, in an age of austerity concerning public health for most countries (developed and developing)—investment in public health surveillance to feed into global surveillance networks may not produce the greatest local, national or global health benefit.

In terms of local engagement, we observed the fundamental importance of local capacity to act on surveillance. The capacity to act on surveillance informs the level of transparency that a government will abide by in outbreak response (as with pandemic influenza preparedness in Chapter 3 and a pandemic outbreak event in Chapter 2); it also affects the level of trust the public will have in their government's competence to respond to individuals rights and needs (Chapter 1), while mitigating the spread of the outbreak amongst the population (Chapter 4). However, there is an underlying equity issue concerning the level of investment states are to make to ensure their public health systems are responsive to global surveillance alerts, and in accommodation of different levels of national capacity and income. Chapter 8 highlights this most markedly in the sense that while the Indonesian government did not reject the need for global surveillance, they did reject the inequity that followed their compliance with surveillance—the loss of control over the income and product to be defended against avian influenza. This was unprecedented, but we would contend that it largely occurred because the Indonesian government expected that its cooperation would deliver local benefit. When Indonesia's compliance did not lead to the expected benefit, it used the only leverage available to it by withholding the virus. As such, we agree with the authors in Chapter 10 who warned that a failure to connect health equity with health capacity is a risk that global surveillance alerts and response will struggle to address and have ongoing outbreak containment ramifications.

As we identified in Chapter 1, global surveillance originated from a desire to protect trade and travel, but it also derived from a desire to protect individual's health, which in turn facilitates collective opportunity to engage in trade and travel. For individuals to freely trade and travel they must have the economic and personal freedom to do so—without fear of persecution. As the H1N1 and Zombie outbreaks (chapters 2 and 4, respectively) highlighted—while global surveillance is to take into account the affect of surveillance alerts on the rights of individuals (Chapter 1)—its effects cannot always be managed. Citizenship, ethnicity and the disease itself produce markers of difference that will make certain groups vulnerable—global surveillance may produce action to prevent the spread of disease but it can also stigmatize and publicize those affected in ways that these individuals cannot control. The revised IHR goes a long way, in comparison to its predecessor, in acknowledging the need for those conducting surveillance to be mindful of their obligations to recognize and abide by human rights frameworks, but this also requires sensitive attunement to the political situation in states that are being surveyed. The technical discussions in chapters 5 and 6 highlighted how the political role of technical surveillance is regarded as a second order priority to the technical and medical benefit from surveillance. Politics must be overcome to achieve the advances of surveillance. This view has been replicated beyond network surveillance providers, as evidenced in discussions concerning the necessity for a US National Strategy for Biosurveillance (Chapter 9). Technical providers may be naïve concerning the potential political influence of heightened global surveillance capacity, or they may be acutely aware and wish to keep this influence or underplay it to facilitate their work. In the case of governments who are enthusiastic (see Chapter 5 on G8 GHSAG and Chapter 9 on US' National Strategy for Biosurveillance), voiced enthusiasm for global surveillance consistently fail to mention how extreme differences in surveillance and diagnostic capacity between countries can be accommodated to strengthen domestic action (as highlighted in Chapter 10).

The integration of surveillance into the public health system has probably received the greatest amount of focus in the literature. Assisting states with IHR compliance and managing IHR compliance with competing health priorities in strained public health systems have both been the subject of discussion and analysis since the revisions were passed in 2007. However, as Chapter 3 highlights, what this actually requires states to do upon notice of the first alert remains somewhat of a mystery. Is the first alert of a novel influenza strain predicting the next global pandemic influenza, or is it just identifying an anomaly that will be contained with effective public health risk management? That question of how to integrate surveillance alerts into action that manages risk and produces resilience without panic is as much a political calculation as it is a public health exercise that frequently proceeds on a case-by-case "work in practice."

Finally, the chance to appeal surveillance is in many respects the default against all of the above. When all else fails, the chance to appeal to authorities outside of a failed government response, or a failed international response, is vital. Up to this point, we have observed it work in different ways. For governments, it is often humiliation and defeat as we saw by those officials whose careers were affected due to their actions during the SARS outbreak in China in 2003, and the Swine Flu outbreak in USA in 1976. For the international system, this right to appeal may produce a situation where WHO finds its own authority being challenged. This could have ramifications for whether member-states have trust and faith in WHO's advice in future outbreak events.

At the end of Chapter 2, Rushton and Kamradt-Scott outlined how the H1N1 case demonstrated that few outbreaks can be kept "quiet" these days. Outbreak control is affected by the discourse that surrounds these events. Outbreaks carry political baggage, and as we have highlighted, this baggage has risen to a global level. Everyone can now observe and judge failure to respond to an outbreak over a 24–48 hour window. We can even judge silence as a failure thanks to the proliferation of systems available to pick up outbreak "noise" (chapters 5 and 6). As such, global surveillance is as much a political act with political consequences as it is a technical one. It must be responsive to individual and multi-actor expectations. This is the politics of surveillance that must be kept in mind as much as the progression of its technology and involvement of multiple actors.

Next Steps

The chapters in this volume demonstrate just how much disease surveillance systems have matured and become vital to the international community. Surveillance is at the core of global strategies to stop any future pandemics in their tracks before they can cause too much illness and death. It has encouraged a proactive stance and intense attention previously unseen and largely considered unsustainable just a short while ago. That does not mean, though, that there exists no room for improvement. The analysis presented in these chapters also point to new areas that remain underspecified or underexplored at this time. As disease surveillance goes forward and comes to play an even more integral role in international politics and global health, academics and policymakers will need to seriously grapple with four key issues.

First, there has been relatively little attention paid to how and whether the various disease surveillance systems are integrated with one another. As it currently stands, each system largely operates autonomously, relying on its own algorithms, analysts, and information sources. To a certain extent, this makes sense. Different systems have different strengths, tapping into different language communities and demonstrating different sensitivities to various anomalous reports. This allows for a measure of competition that could help foster innovation, as well as offer governments and international organizations a greater diversity of information sources. The different systems could potentially backstop each other, decreasing the likelihood that the international community will overlook a potential disease outbreak. That said, these same strengths could ultimately undermine the efficacy of these systems. Too many systems presenting too much information could lead to a cacophony of signals that overwhelm policymakers or inadvertently drown out important warnings. There is such a thing as too much information, and it would be unwise to trust that policymakers who may have little direct experience with public health or disease surveillance have the skills and expertise necessary to cut through the noise to find the right signal. This possibility raises questions about how and whether the various disease surveillance systems could work together to harness the power of their different strategies while avoiding a situation where policymakers get overwhelmed by information. Davies (2012) and Wenham (Chapter 8) both demonstrate that disease surveillance systems can work together, but they also show how these collaborations can fall victim to changes in international organization structures or disagreements among surveillance systems. The importance of addressing the possibility of collaboration and integration will only grow as more systems come online in the coming years.

Second, many of the disease surveillance systems that have become prominent in recent years exist outside formal governmental control. Some draw on national and international government resources more explicitly, while others have only tangential connections to formal government structures. Given the potentially intrusive nature of disease surveillance systems and their importance for encouraging or discouraging particular government actions, the ambiguous connections to the rights and legal protections offered by governments become problematic. To whom does a person make an appeal or lodge a complaint if a non-governmental entity fails to respect rights? Are these disease surveillance systems, which operate in multiple countries, subject to the privacy laws that exist in various countries? The same system may operate in many countries, but the subjects of that system's surveillance could have radically different rights and legal protections. This raises questions about whether the IHR and other treaties and agreements that have empowered disease surveillance systems need to be more explicit about the rights of appeal available to subjects. International law has empowered disease surveillance systems and made them important tools in the global health arsenal, but it has not explicitly considered the international intersection of privacy rights and disease surveillance.

Third, serious questions remain about how the benefits of disease surveillance systems will be distributed. The Indonesia virus sharing case may have ultimately reached a resolution point, but it is symptomatic of potential future conflicts. It is too cavalier to assert that everyone around the world benefits from improved disease surveillance. There clearly exists a very real sense in some developing countries that disease surveillance systems largely benefit wealthier states. The rich countries can afford the drugs to combat the illnesses discovered by these systems and the infrastructure necessary to establish and maintain surveillance networks. Surveillance gives wealthy states time to prepare, while few poor states can verify a novel outbreak of encephalitis, for example, from their annual caseload. Even though the IHR require all states establish disease surveillance systems, they provide no resources to assist states with the action that must follow such an undertaking—diagnostic capacity to verify the outbreak. Nor is it certain states see it in their interest to spend their finite finances on a surveillance infrastructure that will seemingly benefit wealthier governments. Smith describes surveillance systems as luxury goods, and actions by some governments would suggest that they would agree with his analysis. This means that the international community must figure out how to create a system whereby there is a more equitable distribution of surveillance's benefits. Disease surveillance is only as strong as the weakest link, and a state that perceives little benefit to such a system is unlikely to be a strong link in the chain. Furthermore, there needs to be a greater exploration of the intersection between surveillance's benefits and private industry, particularly the pharmaceutical industry. As chapters 9 and 10 illustrates clearly, distrust of surveillance systems can arise when private interests are seen as being privileged over developing states. Was this an anomalous situation due to Indonesia's unique political circumstances, or is it part of a larger indictment of the accrual of surveillance's benefits to pharmaceutical companies in developed states?

Finally, the global health community has started to pay increasing attention to noncommunicable diseases like cancer, heart disease, and stroke. These disease cause more illness and death than infectious diseases, but they receive far less attention from executive levels of government. Disease surveillance systems are generally calibrated to find and track outbreaks of infectious illnesses. Can the same techniques be applied profitably toward noncommunicable diseases? Should they? Does the increased attention paid to NCDs distract from focusing on diseases that have historically been more the target of surveillance efforts, like tuberculosis and HIV/AIDS? In 2014 we remain in a situation where, despite all this technology, more than half of the World Health Assembly member-states fail to consistently collect health data from birth to death. Global disease burden datasets are mostly calculated assumptions. Given the presumed disease burden coupled with collective knowledge gaps, there is a need to think about creative uses of surveillance technology beyond infectious disease alerts. In discussions on the next phase of universal development goals after the conclusion of the Millennium Development Goals in 2015, the focus on health has increasingly turned to universal health care coverage (Rottingen et al. 2014). For a number of states, the relationship between universal health care coverage and the containment of communicable *and* noncommunicable disease is vital to improve political responsiveness to progress health outcomes for all. How would surveillance be enhanced in an environment where every state commits to some form of universal health care coverage? What is clear is that the focus, attention and response of many actors explored in this volume would change if this goal were achieved beyond 2015. As such, global surveillance networks do not solve the outbreak response puzzle but they do enhance to discussions about the optimal environment to overcome knowledge gaps in the area of public health data, and democratization of technology. These health technology initiatives are, as we have sought to demonstrate, intrinsically political. Technical advances and proficiencies are vital but so too is ensuring that the political framework is in place to build improved disease outbreak databases and responses.

Reference

Davies, Sara E. (2012), "Informal Disease Surveillance Networks," *Global Change, Peace and Security*, Volume 24, Issue 1, 2012.

Røttingen, John-Arne (lead author) for Working Group on Health Financing (2014), *Shared Responsibilities for Health: A Coherent Global Framework for Health Financing*, Chatham House Report, May. http://www.chathamhouse. org/sites/files/chathamhouse/field/field_document/20140521HealthFinancing.pdf.

Index